The Hip Mama
Survival Guide

Yo Mama's Daybook

Sunday	Monday	Tuesday	Wednesday
	1 Volunteer planting flowers at kids school. Go home to find 48-hour electricity notice.	**2** Call and plead with electricity company. Take baby to doctor, refrain from flirting with pediatrician. Wonder if this is dysfunction.	**3** Buy organic rocket espresso to help battle chronic sleep deprivation. Whine about job prospects. Guilt-trip ex-boyfriend into paying electricity bill.
7 Kids to various fathers for visits. Try to catch up on work, end up vegging with *People* magazine and gallon of ice cream. Puke. Definitely pregnant again.	**8** Write nasty emails to president@ whitehouse.gov, get "auto-reply." Buy new clothes for family court.	**9** Spend all day in family court waiting for case to come up, feel like watching Jenny Jones. Work all night.	**10** Buy more rocket espresso. Paint car with kids.
14 Kids go to various fathers for visits. Beach party—tan stretch marks.	**15** Cut neighborhood kids' hair like Ernie and Bert's. Go to three job interviews. Forget to wear bra or shoes.	**16** Do pirate radio show, some guy calls in to rant about the "breakdown of the American family." Click.	**17** Stage "Welfare reform" protests at state capitol. Get ticketed for "illegal assembly." Stress out when kids ask if police are "good guys or bad guys."
21 Kids go to various fathers for visits. Go to zine-fest, tell publisher of "Pastrami Nation" that he has all together too much time on his hands.	**22** Go to new temp job. Co-workers call Newt "our boy." Try not to scream out loud.	**23** Buy rocket espresso. Work 'til 2 A.M. Kids wake up at 2:30 A.M.	**24** Try to join YMCA, get told that financial assistance applications take two months to "process."
28 Kids to various fathers for visits. Sleep for 18 hours straight.	**29** Lash out at co-workers who call New "our boy," get reprimanded for discussing politics on the job. Plan a long vacation.	**30** Call landlord and beg for rent mercy. Teach kids how to do pirate radio—they play Nina Hagen and simulate alien take-over of station.	**31** Accept the fact that we live in a chaotic universe. Wonder if it's all dysfunction.

Thursday	Friday	Saturday
4 Hear that flowers at school have been trampled, have "cycle of life and death" discussion with kids. Cancel therapy. Buy pregnancy test instead.	**5** Find myself watching Jenny Jones at 2 A.M.—remember that I have a few things to be thankful for (like that's not me getting yelled at on the show).	**6** Take kids to farmer's market. Play Monopoly Jr. all afternoon— go bankrupt. 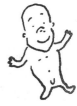
11 Do 15 loads of laundry while the kids play with clay in the kitchen. Try to clean clay off kitchen ceiling. Cancel therapy. Try to quit drinking coffee.	**12** Apply for seven jobs. Write four articles. Buy toilet paper.	**13** Take kids to Ani DiFranco show, try to explain to kids why it is socially acceptable for rock stars to cuss. 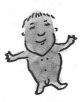
18 Go to kids' art show opening— notice that family law attorney and babysitter are in family portrait. Go to therapy and ask if this is dysfunction, therapist skirts question.	**19** Go to four more job interviews. Forget to take out facial piercings.	**20** Take kids to farmer's market, 6-year old says we don't eat enough brussel sprouts. Wonder if this is dysfunction.
25 Mom comes over to babysit. Wants to know how children got clay on the kitchen ceiling. Cancel therapy.	**26** Stage protest against instant formula marketing at local hospital. Get ticketed for "illegal stopping." Stress out when kids ask if doctors are "good guys or bad guys."	**27** Ask kids what they plan to do over spring break. One says "Rob the President and take over the White House." Wonder if this is dysfunction. 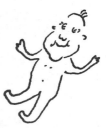

The Hip Mama Survival Guide

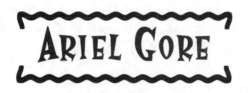

ARIEL GORE

Advice from the Trenches on . . .

Pregnancy • Childbirth • Cool Names • Clueless Doctors •
Potty Training • Toddler Avengers • Domestic Mayhem • Support
Groups • Right-Wing Losers • Work • Day Care • Family Law •
The Evil Patriarchy • Collection Agents • Nervous Breakdowns •
And WAY More

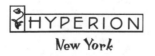

HYPERION
New York

The information contained in this book is not intended to be a substitute for medical advice. Consult your physician or certified nurse-midwife for advice on pregnancy.

Illustrations by Mary Lawton

Gore, Ariel
    The Hip mama survival guide: advice from the trenches on: pregnancy, childbirth, cool names, clueless doctors, potty training, toddler avengers, domestic mayhem, support groups, right-wing losers, work, day care, family law, the evil patriarchy, collection agents, nervous breakdowns, and way more / Ariel Gore.
      p. cm.
   ISBN 0-7868-8232-8
   1. Mothers—United States.   2. Motherhood—United States   3. Child rearing—United States.   4. Parenting—United States.
   I. Hip mama   II. Title.
   HQ759.G629   1998
   306.874'3—dc21   97-33291
                         CIP

Book design by Christine Weathersbee

First Edition

10 9 8 7

hip 1. *adj. slang*: Aware; Informed. **2.** *n.* The part of the human body projecting below the waist on either side, formed by the upper femur. **3.** *n.* A place where young children sit when tired of walking. **4.** *n.* The fruit (red when ripe) of a wild rose. **5.** Whatever you want it to be.

mama 1. *n.* Mother, informal. [repetition of the infantile sound ma] **2.** *n.* One who has a maternal relationship to, nurtures, puts up with, teaches, encourages, constructively yells at, heats from a can or makes chicken soup for, is available for long talks with, and/or generally makes it her (his) business to take care of the next generation. **3.** *n.* A quality or condition that gives rise to another. **4.** *n.* One who loves her children fiercely and herself unconditionally.

TEN FACTS EVERYONE SHOULD KNOW ABOUT MOTHERING

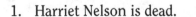

1. Harriet Nelson is dead.

2. Small families do not need minivans.

3. Nervous breakdowns are usually temporary.

4. Stretch marks fade.

5. Nuclear families are fast becoming the minority.

6. Motherhood will change you, but you can still be yourself.

7. It doesn't cost a million dollars to raise a kid.

8. You can nurse, even after nipple-piercing.

9. It is not nice to name a child Cappuccino.

10. If you do it anyway, she will change her name to Jill.

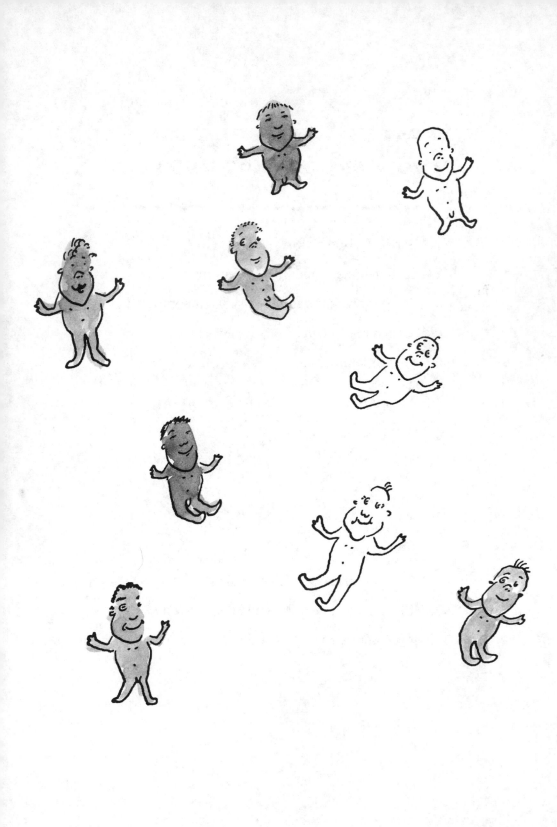

CONTENTS

Introduction ~~~~~~~~~~~~~~~~~~~~~~~~~ 1

PART ONE:
FROM HERE TO MATERNITY

Chapter 1   In the Beginning ~~~~~~~~~ 11
Are You Ready for Mamahood?
Your Body Becomes an Apartment
Hip Mama Boot Camp
Your Average First Trimester
Your Average Second Trimester
Your Average Third Trimester
The High-Risk Pregnancy
The Hip Mama Layette
The Hip Mama Comfort Kit
Preventive Family Law
Rebel Mom: Allison Abner

Chapter 2   Childbirth Sucks ~~~~~~~~~ 41
Childbirth Denial
Home Birth
How Your Labor Might Go
What's the Deal with Medical
   Intervention?
Your Birth Plan
The Best-Laid Plans:
   Dealing with Disappointments
About Circumcision
Name Calling
Rebel Mom: Julie Bowles

Chapter 3   Hey, Baby ————————————68

    Culture Shock
    How Crazed Are You?
    Kicking Back
    Getting Help
    You Can Nurse, Even After Nipple-Piercing
    Mother Earth or Mother Sanity: The Diaper Debate
    To Immunize or Not to Immunize
    Unless You're Ready for Another Babe . . .
    Rebel Dad: Glen Bergers

PART TWO:
THE CHAOS THEORY OF PARENTING

Chapter 4   Toddler Avengers ———————87

    The Screaming Mad Hullabaloo
    Closing the Milk Bar
    Potty Training
    On Rage, Spanking, and the Rest of It
    Rebel Mom: Cherie McCoy

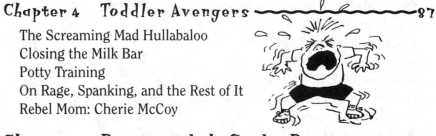

Chapter 5   Beauty and the Gender Beast ————106

    Point Out the Bearded Lady
    Free Polly Pocket
    Negotiate a Testosterone Truce
    Decolonize Your Brain
    Tell the Ad Wizards Where to Go
    Do as You Say
    Rebel Mom: Mary Kay Blakely

Chapter 6   Finding Your Village ————————123

    Don't Even Think About Staying Home with the Curtains Drawn
    Old Friends, New Friends
    Support Groups
    Co-op Parenting
    Rebel Mom: Jessica Mitford

Chapter 7 "Family Values"————————135

Check Your "Family Values" IQ
What's a Girl to Do?
The Dreaded "Familia Nervosa"
Labels to Make You Feel Bad
Why No One Ever Wins the "Debate"
Apocalypse Parenting
If Yo Mama Were President
Rebel Mom: Judith Stacey

Chapter 8 Work and School in the Land of Motherhood————————157

Nine to Five
Know Your Rights, Ladies
I Hate My Job!
Back to School with Baby
False Starts
Rebel Mom: Wendy DeJong

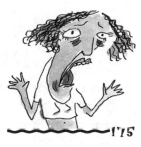

PART THREE: MAJOR BUMMERS

Chapter 9 Nervous Breakdowns (Are Usually Temporary)————————175

"What Is Happening to Me?"
Getting Help
Art and Psyche
And Now a Word from
  New Age White-Light Girl
"I've Been Unexpectedly Called Away"
Redesigning Your Life
Rebel Mom: Tamar Spiegelman-Kern

Chapter 10 Poverty Without Despair —————192

Buying Time
Confessions of a Collection Agent
The Art of Denial
Finding Outside Resources
Child Support
Rebel Mom: Shamama Motheright

Chapter 11 Surviving Family Breakup —————231

Emergency Action
Avoiding Evil Judges and Hard-Ass Attorneys
Adventures in Family Court
Helping Our Kids Through
The Long Haul
Rebel Mom: Opal Palmer Adisa

PART FOUR:
BECOMING THE MAMA YOU ARE

Chapter 12 Guerrilla Mothering —————289

A Place Called Tenacity
Don't Shoot
Protection and Overprotection
Taking Leave
Rebel Mom: Susie Bright

Chapter 13 Imperfectly —————242

Survival Notes —————248

Index —————260

THE HIP MAMA
SURVIVAL GUIDE

INTRODUCTION

The same week I started working on this book, I got a call from a researcher at The Family Channel who was totally psyched to book me as a guest on the *Home and Family Show*. All I had to do was send him a few copies of *Hip Mama*—the parenting zine I publish—and he'd pitch the idea to his producers.

I sent off the zines, exchanged a few more phone calls with the researcher, and within a couple of weeks I was scheduled to appear on the show. They'd fly me and my daughter to Los Angeles, put us up in a hotel, and interview me about parenting on live national television. A final preinterview with the segment producer would be necessary, of course, but these things are no big deal.

The producer in question called me a few days later, and we chatted about the zine, about family and politics, and about my plane tickets, which were, he assured me, "in the mail."

I waited and waited but, mysteriously, no tickets arrived. Finally I called the researcher. He seemed as baffled as I was about the missing tickets and asked me to hold the line.

"Well," he said when he picked up the phone again a moment later. "They decided not to do the segment, apparently because of your political views. . . . This is The *Family* Channel. You know what that means, don't you?"

Not being a Family Channel viewer, I didn't know. (If I had, I might have kept my liberal mouth shut until the cameras were rolling.)

The researcher transferred me to the producer.

"Oh, Ariel," he said cheerfully. "I've been meaning to call you. We overbooked this week. We'll have to reschedule and get back to you."

"That's funny," I said, just as cheerfully. "I heard that it was for political reasons."

"Well," he admitted, "I agreed with a lot of what you were saying, but you go against this network's mentality. This is The *Family* Channel. You know what that means, don't you?"

"No."

"It's owned by Pat Robertson."

"Oh," I said, finally catching on. "I get it. The *Family* Channel."

"Yeah," he said. "The *Family* Channel."

Silly me. In my excitement over an all-expense-paid trip to Hollywood, I completely forgot that "Family" no longer refers to a group of people who love each other but to something a little more limited like, say, a wealthy white Christian Republican heterosexual married nuclear group of people who may or may not love each other. And I'm just some chick who got herself knocked up a few years back.

How I got booked on Pat Robertson's network in the first place, I will never know, but my little phone adventure with the staff of the *Home and Family Show* pretty well sums up my life as a mom. My daughter and I are a family, but we are not, according to Mr. Robertson and his friends, a capital-F *Family*. And while the book you are about to read is all about family, rest assured, it will never be featured on The *Family* Channel.

Having said this, welcome to *The Hip Mama Survival Guide*—the first real guide to all the madness and grace of parenting the millennial generation.

Millennial. That's what they're calling our kids' generation. There's something dramatic and auspicious about this distinction, if you ask me. Just look at the folks born at the last turn of the century. That generation included Zora Neale Hurston, Margaret Mead, Mao Zedong, Amelia Earhart, Alfred Hitchcock, and Louis Armstrong. The last millennial generation brought us more Incas than ever before in Peru, the Vikings who reached America, and the folks who invented movable type in China. Who knows what kind of adults our kids will grow into, but given the fact that we are raising them in such often-outrageous political times, and in so many new and unconventional ways, they're sure to be an interesting bunch. In the meantime, we get to hang out with them in all their crazy-making delightfulness, and, with some luck, together we will not only survive but we'll be able to laugh a little while we're at it.

It's been said that every generation reinvents motherhood, but one of the cool things about us—the parents of these millennial kids—is that we ourselves come from several different generations. Were you weaned on the cheesy perfection of *Ozzie and Harriet* (which probably makes you a boomer)? *The Brady Bunch* (definitely a slacker)? Or did you belong to that June Cleaver in-between crowd? Whichever make-believe families fueled the maternal dreams and nightmares of your youth, we're all reinventing motherhood together now, and it's no easy task.

Six years before I got that call from the *Home and Family Show*, I gave birth to a gorgeous, mushy-faced baby in an Italian hospital. I didn't know the word for "push" (it's *spingere*, in case you're wondering) and I knew very few other moms with whom I had a language, a generation, or anything else in common.

Even when I moved back to California and rented an apartment in the suburbs with my new baby, the other moms on my cul-de-sac commented that my tattoo, my ripped jeans, my full load of college classes, and my boot-legged riot grrl tapes were, well, something less than motherly. "Your family is so . . . unique," they would say, feigning politeness. Or, "Oh . . . you're her mother? I always figured you were a baby-sitter, you look so young."

They might not have tried to act so polite if they had realized that I really was as young as I looked, that my small family survived on food stamps and welfare, or that I wasn't just-divorced—I had never married.

Logic told me that, among the millions of moms in the world, I couldn't be *that* unique. But the other families in my neighborhood always looked so much more TV-like than mine did. And to make matters worse, the parenting guides at the local bookstore only seemed to confirm the idea that I was, perhaps, a total freak of nature.

It took a long time to realize that I wasn't alone—not by any stretch of the imagination.

In the first few years of Maia's life, as we moved around between suburbs and cities, I slowly began to meet other moms I could relate to. We hung out with our kids and shared stories about parenting in chaos. We were intent on preserving our own identities instead of always being "mommy." We told jokes and commiserated about how we potty-trained our kids or how we learned to ignore the Republicans. We ranted about Barbie dolls, nervous breakdowns, and impossible budgets. Most of all, we assured each other that we weren't totally blowing it—because in parenting, as in horseshoes and dancing, "close enough" counts.

"Wait till summer so she can just run around with no pants on. She'll get sick of having accidents in a few days and she'll use the toilet," my friend Julie told me one winter morning when I was trying, unsuccessfully, to get Maia to sit on her new potty.

"Summer?" I asked, horrified as I remembered the three-year deadline I'd read about in a parenting magazine.

"It's not like she's gonna graduate from high school in diapers," Julie assured me. And she was right. In the whole scheme of things, the fact that Maia wore diapers until she was three and a half was hardly monumental.

Even when the serious shit did happen, the trauma was usually followed by a comforting revelation that the perfect mom-and-apple-pie existence I had imagined when I was pregnant really was a Big Lie.

One of my scarier days as a mama happened when Maia had just turned four and we got a visit from a short, pudgy social worker with a Child Protective Services badge. Someone had called to report that my house was messy, and this lady wanted to check it out. As she stood at the door waiting for my response, I started imagining everything that I ever could have done wrong as a mother. Frozen with panic, I was sure the social worker was going to take Maia away, haul me off to bad-mother jail, and call the six o'clock news to come film my laundry pile. "In this filthy Oakland apartment . . ." the newscaster would begin, monotone.

When I finally managed to speak, I invited the social worker in and tried to act surprised yet confident as she read me the report and checked my freezer, fridge, and closets. Although I passed inspection, I was pretty sure a visit from the county was an experience I was supposed to be ashamed of. This one would certainly render me "unique." So after sitting on my couch and rocking back and forth like a catatonic mental patient for some time after she left, it was with more than a little embarrassment that I finally started calling friends to rant about the ordeal.

The first mom I talked to was, predictably, bewildered. "That's like who comes when you're a child abuser," she reminded me.

But as I talked to more friends, I discovered that fully half of them had been visited by CPS—otherwise known as the Committee for Parental Scrutiny. Fully half. And I was *not* hanging out with a gang of child abusers. Pissed-off ex-husbands and bored neighbors were generally presumed to be the sources of the complaints against our families. And being very lucky as well as relatively good parents, nothing much came of the official visits.

In any case, learning that the only difference between me and half the other moms running around was that I had a big mouth and felt the need to tell everyone about my life traumas did make me feel a whole lot better. It was like looking around the high school locker room and, for the first time, realizing that no one else looked like the anorexic models in fashion magazines either—except maybe the babe changing at the end of the row, and we never really did like *her* anyway.

Around the time I became obsessed with this new locker room realization, I was sitting in my friend Julie's kitchen and flipping through some cheesy national parenting magazine (one that features Pat Robertson–style *Families* rather than families). As we ranted about this and that, an idea started to form.

"We should make a real parenting magazine," I said. "The kids in the pictures would be covered with spaghetti sauce and the moms would be all grunged out." We laughed. But even then it was clear that this was one of those ideas that wasn't going to go away. It was the beginning of my last year of college, and I had to come up with a senior project before they'd let me graduate anyway. So, that night in Julie's kitchen, with her baby covered in spaghetti sauce and the older kids refusing to dry off from their hose fight before dinner, *Hip Mama*, the parenting zine, was conceived.

Telling the truth about mothering would eventually get me dubbed "conservative America's worst nightmare" in dozens of newspapers around the country, but first I had to clear the idea with my thesis advisers at school. When I knocked on their office doors a few days later, I was sure they were going to tell me to get serious if I had any hopes of getting a degree. But because they thought the idea was cool, or because they felt sorry for me standing there with a scruffy toddler, or because it was near the end of the day and they wanted to go home, my advisers smiled and nodded and told me to have the first issue done in four months.

By December, with the help of a little gang of writers, photographers, poets, illustrators, graphic designers, proofreaders, and printers (as well as the college newspaper's computers), I had six boxes of issue number one.

We started giving them to friends, selling them at local bookstores, and sending copies off to newspapers in hopes of getting a little review. There were only 500 copies of that first issue but, almost immediately, I started getting phone calls and little notes in the mail. And they weren't all from my grandmother's friends.

I had imagined, at first, that *Hip Mama* readers would look a lot like me: young, single, poor, maybe urban, academic. But as the letters and phone calls started coming in from around the country, I realized that *Hip Mama* had tapped into something bigger. The community that began to grow, and continues to grow, around the zine is a motley mix of parents. A united front against the "family values" crowd, if you will. We are married, single, and partnered. We range in age from fourteen to sixty-four. We are city girls, suburbanites, and country folks. We are gay, straight, and bi. We come from every background imaginable. We are black, brown, peach colored, and every hue in between. But in spite of all our differences, we have the basics in common: We know our rights; we enjoy our kids; we don't identify with Kathie Lee Gifford anymore than we do with the six-foot-tall, ninety-pound supermodels who dominate the pages of women's magazines; and we prefer the real and lived in all its scary imperfection to the glossed over and bogus. In short, our lineage is more Erma Bombeck and Roseanne than Harriet Nelson and June.

When I first thought about writing *The Hip Mama Survival Guide*, I knew it couldn't be an "advice" book in the traditional sense of the word. I knew we didn't need any more "my-way-is-best" tips on parenting. (We get enough of that from strangers in the supermarket.) Instead, we need support. We need information so that we can choose our own ways to parent. We need options. We need something to cheer us up when we feel like we are mothering in hell and something to help us relax when we are sure it is all about to come tumbling down on our heads. We need insights that come from the real and lived. We need something easy to swallow, without the side effects of Prozac. Basically, we need a book that gathers all this together— experience, stories, and advice on surviving the barely survivable.

I never found that book as I pored over the bookstore shelves. So I decided to write it.

In *The Hip Mama Survival Guide*, you'll find an "expert" quoted here and there, but mostly you'll find stories from other moms. Stories that have helped me through and made me laugh. Stories that will, I hope, remind you that you are not alone, and offer a few tools that will come in handy as you invent motherhood all over again.

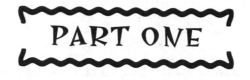
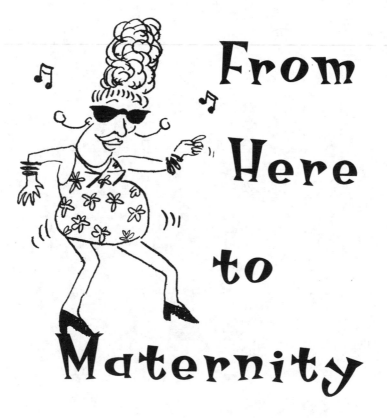

PART ONE

From Here to Maternity

Chapter 1

In the Beginning

*Maybe the rug burns that preceded motherhood will
be worth it after all.*   —Vicky, twenty-nine

The realization that I was totally and completely pregnant came on like a summer storm. The first cloudlike symptoms seemed harmless enough: I woke up one morning and my tits hurt. A few days later I was throwing up paella at the soup kitchen in Valencia, Spain, where I was living with some friends. The nuns gave me strawberry yogurt because I looked so pale, but even when I threw that up, I couldn't be sure. Maybe I was suffering from some bizarre and prolonged case of food poisoning.

It took a couple of weeks before my denial reflex started wearing thin. I began staring at toddlers in the park and watching my boyfriend's face with a new scrutiny—how would our features merge? I gave up going to the soup kitchen altogether and spent my evenings sitting on our terrace. There I counted back the days to my last period, bit my lip, struggled to keep down even a glass of water, and looked up at the sky, which seemed to be growing nearly black with heavy clouds. The storm would certainly come, but the details seemed important. Did my last period start on the day we left Majorca or on the day we arrived? Did I really used to wear a B-cup, or had I been a C-cup all along? And could I have conceived on that night? Or was it that other night? Maybe my period was just late for no reason at all.

As I sat there playing mind games with myself, the little mass of cells that would become my daughter was busy dividing, redividing, and implanting itself on my uterine wall, where it would remain for nine confusing, nauseating months.

I didn't think about my options for very long. I wasn't quite sure why, but I wanted to have a baby. I'd stick around for the storm and hope for the best.

Now, maybe it's just me. Maybe you know why you wanted to be a mom. All I know is that I always imagined I'd have a kid, and then all of a sudden I was pregnant—"like five minutes after I got off the pill," as my friend Molly says—and it felt okay. Excellent, in fact.

Whether the beginning of your long, strange trip to motherhood was marked with a "shit, honey, the condom broke," years of planning and timing and trying, or an ad in *Rolling Stone* that began: *Wanted to adopt . . .* after the pregnancy test or the morning sickness or the phone call that is at once scary and surreal and exciting, we're all out in the same storm—trying to pay attention to the magic, but more conscious of the messy, pain-in-the-ass nature of it all. We wonder if we're really ready, if we have to be *grown-ups* now, if we can really handle being pregnant or waiting for a birth mother to be pregnant for *nine months*. We wonder if we'll be good enough moms, or if we've just completely lost our marbles.

I wish I could tell you that these mixed feelings would eventually come together and flow into a river of pure gratification, but I can't. I can only tell you that the answers to all these questions are probably "yes," and as long as you remember to take care of your own soul throughout your pregnancy, childbirth, and the years of caring so fiercely for your children, your regrets will be fleeting. After all is screamed and done, your life will be a little cooler and a lot more interesting.

Are You Ready for Mamahood?

Is anyone? Not really. But some of us have a little more work to do than others. Just to be obnoxious, I've prepared a quiz to help you analyze your mama potential and alleviate (or confirm) all those worries. You don't have to study for this quiz and, no, you don't have to use a number-two pencil. Just complete the following sentences with the most right-on answer.

1. Eight hours of beauty sleep is:
    a. a necessity.
    b. a blessing.
    c. frivolous; 2 or 3 hours at a stretch is plenty.

2. Turtles, rodents, and lizards belong:
    a. out in the country.
    b. in cages.
    c. running around the house with the rest of the family.

3. Children should be:
    a. not seen and not heard.
    b. seen and not heard.
    c. seen and heard and believed.

4. The thought of sitting on one of those tiny chairs for a parent-teacher conference makes you:
    a. frozen with anxiety.
    b. confused; why is the chair tiny?
    c. slightly tripped out with flashbacks to elementary school, but still functional.

5. Are you prepared to start referring to your mother as "Grandma" and the guy you've been sleeping with as "your father"?
    a. Absolutely not; you'd die first.
    b. No, but you'd be willing to look into "Nana" and "Papa" or some other halfway-there terms.
    c. Why not?

6. Putting on 25 to 50 pounds right now and only expecting to lose, say, half of it, would:
    a. drive you to suicide.
    b. drive you to Jenny Craig.
    c. make you look like a goddess.

7. It's 8 A.M.: the phone is ringing, a baby is crying, there's the faint smell of shit coming from somewhere, Barney's singing at high pitch and high volume, and there's a toy robot in the middle of the room that won't stop repeating "search and destroy, search and destroy . . ." You are:

   a. in the ambulance on your way to the mental ward.

   b. wandering around muttering "I can cope . . ."

   c. in your element and laughing.

8. Pat Robertson is:

   a. God.

   b. Satan.

   c. some dork who's mad at his mother.

9. A clean and orderly home is the sign of:

   a. spiritual and emotional purity.

   b. a weekend of serious housework.

   c. a twisted mind.

10. The word *dilate* refers to:

    a. what your pupils do when you're on certain psychedelic drugs.

    b. a '96 release by Ani DiFranco.

    c. what your cervix will soon be doing.

11. The sound of children laughing makes you:

    a. resentful; how dare they be happy when the world is such a mess?

    b. a nostalgic wreck—such innocence . . .

    c. smile.

12. Your kid is screaming and kicking and convulsing on a tile floor. You are most likely to say:

    a. "Shut up and sit still, you little shit."

    b. "Stop it, you're driving me completely insane."

    c. "I'm going to move you onto the carpet so you don't hurt your head."

Scoring: Give yourself 10 points for every C and 5 points for every B. Your A answers get you nothing, but give yourself 5 bonus points if you already know the difference between "Floam" and "Gack." Add 'em up and check your score.

100–125 points: You go. Are you sure you're not already a mother of six?

60–95 points: You were made for this, girlfriend. Don't worry if you've got a few rough edges. You're well on your way to becoming a fabulous mamawoman.

30–55 points: Okay, so you're a fixer-upper mama. No, really, there's potential here, but we do have a little work to do—prepare for transformation.

10–25 points: Um, have you really considered your options? If you're dead set on the motherhood thing, you might want to invest in some therapy (or perhaps a nanny).

Less than 10 points: Ack! Your fears are justified. Stop. Don't do it! Pawn the baby off on your sister if you have to.

Presuming you're ready for mamahood (or, like most of us, you're totally freaked out and praying like hell), here's a quick run-through of what you can expect if you've got a tenant in your womb. If this doesn't do it for you, there are a surprising number of pregnancy manuals on the market that will give you hundreds of pages of information. I've had the mixed blessing of reading about two dozen of these guides—most are about 300 pages long, contain snapshots taken in the 1970s of pregnant white women with their partners (and with or without heads coming out of their vaginas), and offer pretty good medical and physical information on everything from fetal development to postpartum blues. (See "Survival Notes" for recommended reading.) Since I've only got a few dozen pages, however, we're going to skip the snapshots and go for the highlights.

Waiting for an Adoption

When you are preparing to adopt a baby, you may not have to suffer through the physical hell of pregnancy, but the expectation and uncertainty can be just as extraordinary. Without the baby right there in your tummy, it can be hard to grasp the reality of your impending motherhood, and without the visual cue for your many sometimes-clueless friends and acquaintances it can be hard to convince folks that, *Yes, things are about to change dramatically around here.* As one mama tells me, "People will throw you a baby shower when you're pregnant—even though they realize that anything could happen between now and your due date—and yet when you're going through a pregnancy that is not physically your own, people seem to take a let's-wait-and-see attitude."

Of course the process of adoption is uncertain. I know families who didn't find out about their new babies until a few hours before they came home, and other families whose birth mothers changed their minds. All of this can be tremendously stressful, so it is important that we mother ourselves during the whole process.

One mom who has adopted four children tells me that she was nervous with the first one, but she began to realize that a lot of her fears were from external sources. "My parents and my husband's parents have always been more worried than we were. You know, life is uncertain. I could get hit by a truck today, and yet I get up and go about my business and I don't think about that. If I spent my days saying 'Oh my god, I'm going to get hit by a truck today,' I would of course go completely insane. If I spent my birth mother's pregnancy thinking 'I just know she's going to change her mind,' that wouldn't be useful at all. The chances of that are actually quite slim."

While waiting for an adoption, many moms also find time to really process (if you'll excuse the recovery-culture word) their situations. Sometimes there is a grieving process we need to go through about not having children from our own bodies.

We also need to hook up with other mamas who are in the same boat. "Spend the time taking advantage of all the wonderful adoption resources, and network," suggests Luca, who got both of her children through open adoptions. "You can go to conferences, meet people, and read all of the incredible books and materials that have been written about adoption."

When Luca put an ad in *Rolling Stone*, she ended up fielding a lot of calls, but, she said, "I fell in love with birth mothers as a group of people." When she and her husband finally found their birth mother, the young woman came to stay with the couple for the second half of her pregnancy. "It was at times awkward," Luca admits. "But it was certainly bonding. At some point she asked us what we would do if she changed her mind and we said, as honestly as we could, 'Well, we would be very sad, but we would honor your choice.'"

The birth mothers of Luca's children now visit from time to time, and Luca describes the relationship as "surprisingly wonderful."

Mamas who adopt from women they do not know or women who chose not to be directly involved with the family have different experiences. But as one adoptive mama puts it, "Once we put it out of our minds that our family is supposed to be exactly like someone else's—exactly like a nuclear, biological family, or exactly like a family who did an open adoption, for example—another whole world opens up. This is my child. And she was not born of my body. But believe me, I have stretch marks on my psyche."

Your Body Becomes an Apartment

I've heard pregnancy and childbirth compared to just about every creative endeavor on the planet. Authors say that writing a book is like being pregnant; sculptors say that doing a bronze casting is like giving birth; Oscar winners compare those who helped them make their movies to midwives; and painters talk about their creative process like gestation. So I feel obligated to warn the artists and writers among you mamas-to-be that you are *not* in for a familiar experience. Other than the fact that you are forming something out of nothing, the book-as-pregnancy (or bronze-casting-as-pregnancy or neo-impressionist-painting-as-pregnancy) is a totally bogus metaphor. I've been hammering away at writing various sections of this book for more than a trimester, and I haven't vomited once. Just to double-check, I called a few other writers and artists I know. Sure, they'd used the metaphor, but no one I talked to could think of any actual similarities. That's because, in reality, very few art projects actually make you vomit, cause stretch marks, change the texture of your hair, compel you to love ice cream and hate eggs, or make you wonder if you'll ever be the same person again.

Being pregnant is more like coming down with a case of malaria or intestinal worms.

When my sister and I lived in Hong Kong, we knew a Scottish woman who, after quite a few months on the island, was suddenly convinced that she had contracted some dreaded illness that lurked in the South China Sea. Also convinced that no Hong Kong doctor would know how to treat her ailment, our friend flew to London to see a tropical disease specialist. The British doctors didn't have to do too many tests before they informed her that she was, of course, pregnant.

Alice Walker described her 1969 pregnancy this way: "The first three months I vomited. The middle three I felt fine and flew off to look at ruins in Mexico. The last three I was so big at 170 pounds I looked like someone else, which did not please me." And that pretty well sums it up.

Everyone has their favorite trimester. My friend Dionne preferred the first, when "I knew there was something inside me that no one else could see, like a mystical secret." The most popular trimester is the second, when the storm of emotional chaos and nausea of the first three months has settled down, your belly begins to grow mysteriously full of promise, and the sex is at its best. A few women

I've talked to preferred their last trimester, when, as one mom put it, "Every part of my body was so full, and I felt like a little girl waiting for Christmas. Every day I would think *Will this be the day?* And I would pay attention to everything that happened so I would be able to tell my son *This is what happened the day you were born—the fruit weighed heavy on our plum tree, or my car broke down, or there was an old woman at the flea market who told me that you would be tall, with nice eyebrows."*

Hip Mama Boot Camp

No matter which aspects of your pregnancy end up being your favorite and which make you want to go running and screaming to turn back the clock and double up that damn condom, from the moment you find out you're pregnant, consider yourself enlisted in Hip Mama Boot Camp. Basic training begins with how you treat your body.

If you're like me and you already have to remind yourself on a daily basis that woman cannot live on root beer and licorice alone, then getting used to eating well can be about as easy as dragging your butt to a 7 A.M. dentist appointment every day of the week. But it *is* doable. My psychologist friend tells me that it takes two weeks to break an old habit and twenty-eight days to form a new one, so maybe after that painstaking first moon, you'll be addicted to being healthy.

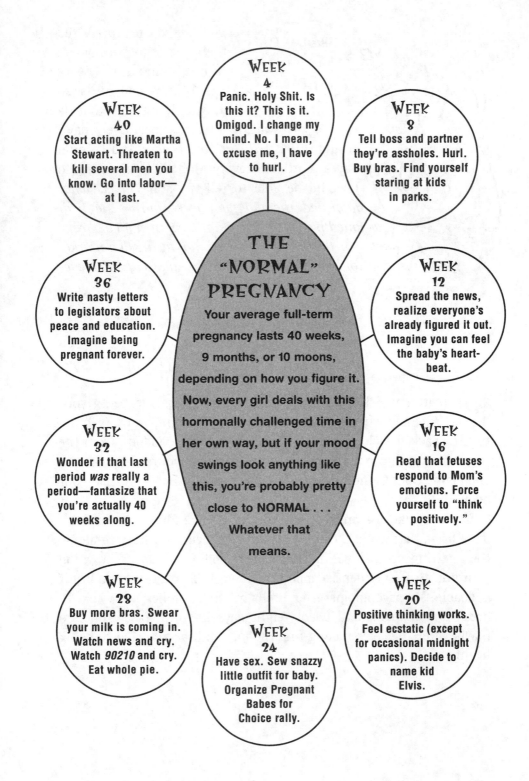

WEEK 4
Panic. Holy Shit. Is this it? This is it. Omigod. I change my mind. No. I mean, excuse me, I have to hurl.

WEEK 40
Start acting like Martha Stewart. Threaten to kill several men you know. Go into labor—at last.

WEEK 8
Tell boss and partner they're assholes. Hurl. Buy bras. Find yourself staring at kids in parks.

THE "NORMAL" PREGNANCY
Your average full-term pregnancy lasts 40 weeks, 9 months, or 10 moons, depending on how you figure it. Now, every girl deals with this hormonally challenged time in her own way, but if your mood swings look anything like this, you're probably pretty close to NORMAL . . . Whatever that means.

WEEK 36
Write nasty letters to legislators about peace and education. Imagine being pregnant forever.

WEEK 12
Spread the news, realize everyone's already figured it out. Imagine you can feel the baby's heartbeat.

WEEK 32
Wonder if that last period *was* really a period—fantasize that you're actually 40 weeks along.

WEEK 16
Read that fetuses respond to Mom's emotions. Force yourself to "think positively."

WEEK 28
Buy more bras. Swear your milk is coming in. Watch news and cry. Watch *90210* and cry. Eat whole pie.

WEEK 20
Positive thinking works. Feel ecstatic (except for occasional midnight panics). Decide to name kid Elvis.

WEEK 24
Have sex. Sew snazzy little outfit for baby. Organize Pregnant Babes for Choice rally.

Generally speaking, you have to be most careful about what you put in your body during the first three months of your pregnancy. This is when the embryo is in "formation" and the baby's little parts are developing. After you start show-ing, you're in the "growth" stage, when all the fetus really has to do is get big and strong. When you find out you're pregnant, please don't spend too much time freaking out about what you may have already put into your system before you realized you were housing your babe-to-be. Talk to your midwife if you have serious concerns, but focus on the here and now. The main trick is to have a healthy, bal-anced diet and to avoid toxins, both natural and unnatural. Check with your midwife about getting some prenatal vitamins with iron (it's easy to become anemic) and vitamin E (it may help your skin).

When I was pregnant I con-sumed some of the things I'm about to tell you not to, as did some of the other women I interviewed for this book. I say this not because I want to make light of the risks, but because I worry about moms' anxiety lev-els. If you have a couple of beers one afternoon, for example, the best thing you can do is accept it and move on. If you're getting

Your Basic Rules of Pregnancy

- Eat a balanced diet.
- Get your prenatal care by making and keeping regular doctor/midwife appoint-ments.
- Chill out as much as possible and get plenty of sleep.
- Avoid immunizations, X rays, and any drugs that are not medically necessary.
- Don't get any new body piercings below the neck.
- Don't handle the cat litter. (Cat poop can be infected with toxoplasmosis, a disease that can harm your fetus).
- Stay active. Check with your doctor or midwife about the kinds of exercise you should be getting, but low-impact activities like walking, dancing, and swimming are good bets.
- Wear your seat belt low.
- Don't hang out with anyone who makes you feel like shit.
- Don't read *Sophie's Choice*. (This last tip came from my mom, who actually sent me a telegram when I was five months pregnant that read, simply, "Don't read Sophie's Choice. STOP. Call your mother. STOP.")

plastered every night, on the other hand, you need to get help. As soon as you think about getting pregnant you lose the right to be self-destructive. Incidentally, you never get this particular right back. It was an adolescent thing—get over it. All that said, here are the basic consumables to avoid while you've got a tenant in your womb:

- **Food that Smells Moldy or Unappealing:** Don't eat anything that doesn't smell appealing to you. When you're pregnant, your sense of smell is naturally heightened so you can detect toxins in foods. If things don't smell fresh to you, don't let your friends convince you that you're bonkers. That "fishy" or moldy smell should be a red flag.

- **Coffee, Tea, and Soda:** If you must have coffee, tea, herbal tea, or cola, you should strictly limit the amount you drink, especially in your first trimester. All the caffeine and other natural toxins will just make you—and your babe—ill.

- **Alcohol:** Alcohol can cause serious birth defects and retardation, and it is responsible for several thousand cases of fetal alcohol syndrome in the United States each year. There is no established safe daily dose of alcohol for pregnant women, but studies have found that more than one drink a day increases the risk of mild to serious mental impairment.

- **Cigarettes:** I could use this whole book to list the reasons why it's not a good idea to smoke while you're pregnant, but here are the highlights: smokers have lower-weight and more premature babies; smoking inflicts tons of toxins on the placenta and embryo and makes your fetus feel anxious; smoking diminishes your sense of smell and taste, which would otherwise help you avoid harmful foods; and smoking depletes your bloodstream vitamin C. If that isn't bad enough, after the baby is born nicotine will get into your breast milk and leave your baby addicted. If you're a smoker, quit. At the very least, cut down on the number of cigarettes you smoke, take vitamin C supplements, and pick up a copy of *Protecting Your Baby-to-Be* by Margie Profet to get a full report on which foods you would avoid if only you could smell.

- **Legal Drugs:** Only take drugs that are medically necessary, and if you are being prescribed medication (including antibiotics), tell your doctor that you are pregnant. Request an up-to-date list of the over-the-counter drugs that are considered safe for pregnant women. No, you can't take ibuprofen—it's Tylenol (acetaminophen) that you can use sparingly. And the only decongestant you can take is Sudafed.

- **Recreational Drugs:** Do I have to tell you that you can't smoke pot, do cocaine, drop acid, or take any other illegal drugs when you're pregnant? If you are addicted, get treatment immediately and talk to your midwife about the danger you may have already exposed your fetus to. Illegal drugs are especially dangerous because you never quite know what's in them (a little talcum powder here, a little battery acid there). If you are addicted to hard drugs, your baby will be born addicted and go through withdrawal, and Child Protective Services will probably take your baby away. If you use recreational drugs regularly and you are not yet pregnant, talk to your midwife before you try to conceive. This is serious. Don't screw around.

Your Average
First Trimester

Nia calls her trips to the supermarket "white-knuckle experiences." As she pushes through aisle after aisle of nauseating food clutching her shopping cart, the thought of actually getting through the meat department and up to the checkout seems like a monumental task. She finally gets out of the store with her little sack of food, climbs wearily onto the bus, and just as she sits down near the front, she vomits into her handbag. Nia is: (a) drunk as a skunk, (b) suffering from severe supermarket phobia and in need of medication, or (c) in her first trimester. You know it. As one newly pregnant friend puts it, "It's always morning around here."

While you're trying to figure out if you have a tropical disease and whether it's terminal, and you're tripping out over why they call it "morning" sickness when it happens morning, noon, and night, your baby-to-be is a busy little bundle of cells. Just about every week your fetus—or embryo, as it's called during formation—grows some new vital organ. First there's a heartbeat, and it's uphill from there.

What's in Formation?

Week 3	spinal cord and nervous system
Week 4	liver, stomach, intestines, lungs
Week 5	arms and legs
Week 6	diaphragm (no, that's not a method of birth control)
Week 7	measurable brain waves and the embryo's sex becomes apparent (hmmm . . . is there a connection?)
Weeks 8–9	face
Week 10	communication between muscles and brain
Week 11	vocal cords

Even after all this action, though, your baby-to-be is only about the size and weight of a mini Milky Way bar.

In your first three months of pregnancy, you'll probably only gain about three or four pounds, but you can also expect to start relating to Alanis Morissette when she sings "I'm sad but I'm laughing . . ." Add to her list *I'm tired but I can't sleep, I'm constipated but I'm peeing, I'm dizzy and I keep salivating.* Don't be surprised if your appetite increases, you have bizarre food aversions and cravings, your boobs are sore, your areolas (the area around your nipples) darken, and you're struck by heartburn, indigestion, bloating, mood swings, and crying jags. I know all of this sounds like great fun, but think of it as a three-month initiation. The rest of this rite of passage isn't nearly as bad—until labor, that is.

Your Average
Second Trimester

What can I say? The sex is great. Not only can you expect to be totally horny, but the sex itself is awesome. Some women even report having their first orgasms or first multiple orgasms during this glorious season. Rest assured that unless your midwife tells you otherwise, you can have as much sex as you want while you're pregnant, but you may have to get creative with positions as you get bigger, and, of course, you may not want to bother with the missionary position at all.

Intense orgasms can get your contractions going only if you're ready to go into labor, but super-intense-vibrator-induced orgasms can actually send you into premature labor—so be careful with the wand. You should also avoid anal sex, seeing as you're already prone to hemorrhoids when you're in a family way.

Now, I've heard a few stories about men who didn't think pregnant women were sexy. Please don't listen to any of this bullshit. If your man doesn't think you look awesome, he needs therapy, or maybe he should just go fuck himself in another state and leave you alone.

Finally, while you obviously don't have to worry about getting pregnant, safe sex is always a good thing, so get some colored condoms and have fun.

As for outdoor activities, you'll probably be getting desperate for some maternity clothes around this time, and you may notice that most of them are made for Katie Couric wannabes. Unless you can find some hip urban maternity wear outlet, the dresses they try to sell pregnant women can be downright scary. I recommend avoiding actual maternity wear, except for overalls, spandex, and sweats, and going for leggings and big shirts instead. Comfort should be your main goal, so tell anyone who disses your wardrobe to take a big 'lude and get a life.

Other telltale symptoms of the second trimester include edema (swelling of the feet, ankles, and hands), varicose veins, gaining two to six pounds a month, and (yes!) showing. Acquaintances who aren't in the know will begin to catch on and slowly, cautiously at first, they'll ask . . . *are you*? Their greatest fear is that you are going to say "Naw, I just drink a lot of beer," so, if you hate these people, you can have fun making them feel totally mortified for a couple more months.

Depending on your genes and your age, stretch marks may appear on your belly, breasts, and legs. These lovely marks can be purple, white, or dark brown, depending on your skin color, and will eventually fade to translucent. The folks at the cosmetics counter and the health-food store will try to sell you expensive creams and lotions that claim to prevent stretch marks, and I've talked to plenty of people who swear by vitamin E oil and cocoa butter, but that's all bogus. Massaging your skin with oil can be very nice and relaxing, and it may relieve itching, but you can go ahead and come into acceptance—if your skin is prone to stretch marks, you'll get them.

Facing the World

When you tell folks you're pregnant, their response is supposed to be "Congratulations!" Depending on your age, marital status, job, and hairdo, however, some of the usual excitement might be missing from friends' and family members' voices. Instead you might hear "Oh my god!" "Have you really thought about . . . " or even "How could you!" I myself did not hear a sincere "congratulations!" until my grandmother, the queen of etiquette, sent me a postcard in my second trimester.

Your boss and party-girl friends probably will feel a wee bit abandoned. Your mother will probably start feeling a little resentful ("I'm too young to be a grandma!"). And more than a few casual acquaintances will have their own issues they're prepared to dump on you.

But no matter how all these people react to your news, hold your head high and tell them simply "I think 'congratulations' is the word you're looking for."

A funny thing happens when we get pregnant. Everyone and their senator thinks they can start sticking their nose in our business (or poking our bellies with their fingers) and making all kinds of judgments. This strange and, if you ask me, rude behavior continues right through our careers as mamas. So the time to stop caring what other people think is now.

If you have a pierced belly button you should take the ring out, but you can leave a nipple ring in as long as it feels comfortable. The nice folks at Body Manipulations in San Francisco advise their clients to "listen to their bodies" and act accordingly. If you need to remove rings, you can get a monofilament (translation: littlepiece of plastic fishing line or Weed Eater line) to put through the hole so it won't close up during your pregnancy. While you may not have gotten your piercings from a reputable studio, it's important to go to one for the monofilament and any other maternity piercing needs—this is no time to get an infection. While you don't have to remove clit or labia rings until you go into labor and can, technically, put them back in as soon as the baby is born, I'd consider taking them out early and kissing those piercings good-bye. There's going to be plenty of action down there without having to worry about additional metal and holes. You can always get them redone after you're finished procreating—once you've experienced labor, the pain of repiercing will seem like amateur stuff.

What Your Fetus Is Up To

Weeks 12–15	growing to 13 inches and thumbsucking with newly formed fingers, toes, and tooth buds
Weeks 16–19	moving around noticeably and kickin' ya in the belly
Weeks 20–24	growing a little hair, gripping with hands, able to hear your heartbeat, your voice, and some outside sounds like Nina Hagen's *NunSexMonkRock* at high volume.

Your Average Third Trimester

If you ask me, the third trimester should be spent loafing, dancing, daydreaming, and following that strange nesting urge that compels you to make enough lasagna for a small army and scrub the linoleum in your kitchen with a toothbrush. As the feminist essayist Alta says, "One hesitates to bring children into the world without fixing it up a little. Paint a special room. Stop sexism. Learn to love." With all this to see to, it's a good idea to clear your calendar of all unnecessary doings.

Even if you can't take time off to stop sexism, you'll be plenty busy with heartburn, indigestion, gas, constipation, headaches, shortness of breath, bleeding gums, backaches, and/or leaking breasts. Your boobs will get a lot bigger, as will your belly, and you'll probably notice a heavier, whitish vaginal discharge. If your insides feel all out of whack, it's because your uterus is hogging all the room in your body and your other organs have had to relocate. You'll also have to pee a lot because the fetus will be putting pressure on your bladder.

You should be seeing your doctor or midwife every couple of weeks at this point and making sure that you only hang out with kind people. If possible, you should not be working through the last few weeks, as every task can become a monumental effort—but plenty of moms do work up to the last moment.

As long as your doctor or midwife doesn't go and put you on total bedrest, exercise—such as walking and dancing to a combination of folk rock and hip-hop—may help remind your fetus to get into position and help get your labor going. When you are sleeping, you can prop yourself up with pillows between your legs and behind your back. Spend some time each day on your hands and knees (seriously). Too much sitting while we're driving, working, or vegging can encourage a fetus to stay posterior, which will, in turn, cause the dreaded and very painful back labor.

Last-Minute Fetal Development

Weeks 27–28	eyes open, weighs in at about 2.5 to 5 pounds, retina is able to receive light, brain forms grooves and indentations, eyebrows and eyelashes develop
Weeks 28–39	fattens up
Weeks 39–40	settles into position (with its head down, one hopes) for its journey through the birth canal and into the world.

The High-Risk Pregnancy

If you're over thirty-five, under twenty, have had a miscarriage and/or numerous abortions, have health problems, or have been exposed to other risk factors, your doctor or midwife may classify your pregnancy as "high risk." All this means is that you will have to get a little more medical attention throughout your pregnancy and be even more vigilant about your diet and exercise.

If you're over thirty-five, your obstetrician will be concerned about birth defects and will recommend tests, tests, and more tests, especially amniocentesis.

Young moms need to watch out for anemia, high blood pressure, and toxemia, all of which are more common among teens. The younger the mother, the greater the risk for premature and low-birth-weight babies. These risks are linked to the fact that, as a teenager, you are still growing yourself and are more likely to be undernourished. You can avoid this by eating well. And in general, take care of yourselves, ladies.

Please remember that even if you are in a high-risk group, the chances that something will go wrong are very slim. Miscarriage in the early months of pregnancy and toxemia in the later months are the most common problems, but even these only occur in about 20 percent of pregnancies. My Italian doctors classified my pregnancy as high risk because they thought I was too young and, later, because they didn't think I was gaining enough weight. They did about 50 million ultrasounds (okay, maybe it was only five) and kept telling me that I should be totally stressed out, but all went well, and it probably will go well for you too. Just make sure you keep up with your prenatal appointments and let your midwife or doctor know if anything is worrying you.

The Hip Mama Layette

"**I**'m going to dress my baby all in black," says Anne Marie. "She'll be the coolest."

Actually, she'll be the messiest. There's a reason that people dress babies in white. First of all, it's really hard to find black diapers, let alone black sleepers. But the main reason new moms don't dress their babies in black is that babies spit up a lot. And spit-up is white.

I guarantee that your life will be much easier if you just go with conventional wisdom on this one:

- 8 white undershirts

- a pair of white longjohns

- 3 light-colored sleepers

- 3 light-colored kimonos

- a dozen white receiving blankets

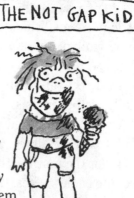

THE NOT GAP KID

There's plenty of room to get creative. Hats, mittens, and booties (presuming your baby will wear them), for example, can be pretty funky. A couple of good nontraditional baby-item sources are Al-Kebu-Lan designs in Los Angeles, reachable at (213) 464-1426, and the National Organization for Women catalog, which you can get by calling (202) 331-0066. Get a couple of hats, a couple of pairs of mittens and booties, and whatever else your heart desires. Knock yourself out on a quilt or blanket too. Get a couple of crib or bassinet blankets and a couple of carriage blankets—this is where that friend with the Martha Stewart heart will come in handy. Make sure someone throws you a shower, and make sure she gets the invitations out a few weeks in advance. If this is your first baby, you'll get just about everything you need at the shower. (Remember to save it all. People are not nearly as generous with babies number two and three.)

Remember to avoid clothes with loose ribbons or strings, tops with flowing sleeves, or zippers that come tight around the neck. I probably don't have to tell you to make sure the stuff is washable and soft. If the phrase "dry clean" was ever in your vocabulary, you can go ahead and delete it now. Feel free to throw away your iron while you're at it too.

Once your kid has a nice little wardrobe, it's on to diapers and bottles. If you're going the cloth route, you'll need about six dozen cloth diapers, six pairs of waterproof pants, six diaper pins, and a couple of plastic pails with lids—or a diaper service. Otherwise get a large box of disposable infant diapers and about a dozen cloth diapers. If you're bottle-feeding, you'll need about fifteen bottles of varying sizes and a sterilization set. If you're breast-feeding (which is easier, cheaper, and healthier), get a couple of bottles and, especially if you're going back to work right away, a breast pump.

Now you've got to stock the bathroom. A few soft baby towels and washcloths, some mild baby soap, baby lotion or oil, A and D Ointment, baby powder, cotton balls, a soft hairbrush, and some baby nail clippers should do the trick.

Finally, it's time to decide where your kid will sleep. I'm not a big advocate of putting them in a crib right away, but having one for later certainly won't hurt.

Unless you are rolling in cash, baby furniture should be borrowed or bought secondhand, except the car seat, which should be new. Changing tables are basically useless—babies can fall off of them, and it's not a big deal to change diapers on the floor—but get one if you must. Most babies I know spent their first few months sleeping in a wicker bassinet, cradle, or a big old baby buggy beside mom's bed. At night, they usually end up right in bed with mom. My daughter slept in a buggy, which, of course, doubled as a stroller and made my life a little easier. A friend of mine recently told me that the buggy was a bad idea—in an earthquake it might roll away. This is paranoia. But, whatever makes mom happy . . .

The Hip Mama Comfort Kit

On to the important stuff: what *you'll* need. Be realistic. You are not going to want to run out to the convenience store at 2 A.M. looking for nursing pads and Pop Tarts. Plan accordingly. Here's what I suggest:

Everyday Wear

- A few pairs of sweats
- A couple of button-down flannel shirts you can nurse in
- A couple of big T-shirts
- Slippers
- Socks
- Nursing bras
- Plenty of underwear

Fem Protection

- Nursing pads
- A bunch of really big sanitary napkins (snag the big blue ones from the hospital if you can)
- Condoms (yes, Virginia, you can get pregnant again)

Kick-Back Gear

- A few mellow but nonlullaby tapes, such as Tracy Chapman, Sweet Honey in the Rock, John Coltrane, or The Cranberries.
- Bath salts
- A few cheesy videos that *will not* make you cry, such as the complete Brady Bunch, *Tank Girl*, or some Bill Murray flick like *What About Bob?*

Consumables

- As much cash as possible earmarked for pizza and other take-out food
- A list of phone numbers for the local restaurants with free delivery
- A couple of frozen lasagnas and a few vats of chicken soup you made when you were in nesting mode (ninth month of pregnancy)
- Some dark beer (as long as you're not in recovery, for relaxation and milk production)
- Tylenol

Add to this list anything else you'll need to chill out for a week or two, and have it all ready and stashed sometime around your seventh month of pregnancy. But please do not stress over your layette or your comfort kit. If you have any friends, they'll call as soon as they hear you've given birth to ask what you need. Tell them to bring food to freeze, to come over and make dinner, to clean the kitchen, or do whatever else you need them to do. These people are not calling to be polite—they really want to come over and see your gorgeous babe. Use them. The excitement dries up all too fast.

Preventive Family Law

For some reason, a lot of people don't think they need to worry about family law until they are in the middle of a crisis. But you shouldn't wait until you get sued for custody to learn the basics about the laws that govern your life as a mom, so this will give you a quick overview.

Family courts vary widely from county to county and state to state, but most are misogynist institutions with little or no understanding of alternative family structures and more interest in patriarchal social engineering than in your individual child's best interest. The English translation of this is that a contested custody case—a case where you or your child's father asks a judge to decide how your family will live—is a nightmare. In many families, however, the nightmare is avoidable.

If given our lives to live over, I can't tell you how many people I've talked to who wish they would have done a little preventive family law *before* their kids were born. To offer you all their insights, I phoned the dozen or so women with the most heinous breakups and custody wars I knew of, thinking I could put together a sort of "Let's Go Hades" for you. Unfortunately, however, most of these moms admit that, at the time, "I was madly in love with him and wanted to spend the rest of my life with him." After a little further questioning, most of them also admitted that "Well, he was a raging alcoholic," or "He did punch me in the stomach when I told him I was pregnant," or some such I-should-have-known. These casual interviews always seemed to end with the same words: "I thought everything would change when the baby was born." Can we end this line of thinking in the world, like, say, RIGHT NOW? Honestly, do you know anyone who knows anyone who turned from an asshole into a prince in nine months? No, I'll venture to say, you do not, and neither do I.

I'm not advocating breaking up with a perfectly cool dude. I'm saying break up with anyone who shows signs of being an asshole. If your asshole-o-meter is impaired (itself a sign that you might be sleeping with one), here are the top-ten signs of asshole-dom:

1. He has *ever* hit you, kicked you, slapped you, pushed you, spat on you, or threatened to hurt you.

2. He drinks and/or does drugs constantly.

3. He irrationally accuses you of having affairs and/or himself disappears for long, unexplained periods of time.

4. He is angry at you for becoming pregnant even though you seem to remember him having something to do with it.

5. He says something about you not going into labor during a certain ballgame and he's not kidding.

6. You feel worse after you spend time with him than you did before.

7. He likes Rush Limbaugh.

8. He tracks all your time and/or your finances.

9. He says he'll hurt himself, you, and/or your children if you leave him.

10. He's gotten into the habit of saying "It will never happen again."

(BONUS TIP #1: It *will* happen again.)

Family advocates also warn that a batterer will often hit his partner for the first time while she is pregnant. Please be aware that this new behavior usually continues throughout the pregnancy and after the baby is born. In other words, run far and fast.

If any of these signs sound familiar, you are likely in an emergency situation and need to see a lawyer and perhaps a counselor, like, yesterday. But even if your partner is not a total dork, a little prenatal law never hurts, and it usually helps.

If you're married when your baby is born, you, your husband, and your child have automatic rights under the law, and both parents have automatic responsibilities. You can hammer out the details of property division in case of a divorce with prenuptial and postnuptial agreements, but custody and child support issues generally cannot be agreed upon ahead of time. If you're not married, it is a really good idea if you can decide, while you are still pregnant, how you want your future family to live. Once you know what you want, you will be able to decide whether you need court orders clarifying your plans. If both parents can agree on a setup, it is best to make a written agreement and file it with the court. If you and your child's father are already at odds, you can talk to a lawyer about whether it is better to take your issues to court or leave well enough alone.

Legal agreements and court orders can change over time, as can your ideas about how you want to raise your child, but having some sort of understanding early on is important. Basically, you are either going to want to ensure that everyone in your family has the same rights as they would if you were married, or you are going to want to limit those rights. It is my humble opinion that whoever carries the baby in her womb should have the biggest say in all of this, but that's not always the way the law works. Be very careful about what you sign. You don't want to limit your maternal rights, and you don't want to listen to a lawyer who's being paid by someone else.

Scary Facts About Family Law

- If parents are not married and there are no court orders, most police departments will take NO ACTION if either parent takes off with the baby.

- It takes a court order to establish paternity if parents aren't married, but the county may file one without your permission if you identify the father in legal documents (e.g., an application for welfare).

- Once paternity is established, the noncustodial parent may have to pay child support, but he is also entitled to visitation with the child.

- In most states, nonbiological lesbian or gay coparents have no legal rights.

- Men win seven out of ten contested custody cases. The reason that most children live with their mothers is that fewer men want custody.

- Batterers are twice as likely to seek custody of their children than nonbatterers.

If you have a complicated situation (more than two adults could claim parentage, for example), you will need to consult with an attorney and get very clean legal agreements signed and filed with your local family court as soon as possible. You can find a family law attorney by calling your local Legal Aid, Commission on the Status of Women, or a women's shelter for a referral. Make sure you get a *family law* attorney who has been practicing for some time in the county where you live. A consultation may be free, but most reasonably priced attorneys charge between $50 and $100 for an initial consultation.

Below are the basics for some common situations. As I write this, the legal information is up-to-date, but laws change, laws vary from state to state, and none of this is meant to take the place of proper legal advice.

Coparenting

Coparenting usually means that two parents share the responsibility for raising their child even though they don't live together. It's sort of the status quo these days for parents who divorce after sharing parental responsibilities within their marriage and who want to keep a similar setup for the kids after they break up. No matter how amicable your relationship with the other parent, however, coparenting is a hard, hard gig. One standard coparenting agreement that works for many parents is for children to live with mom and spend a few afternoons a week with dad when they are babies, and a few weekends a month with dad as they get older.

Single Parenting and Informal Donor Arrangements

If you know you are going to be a single mom, if you got pregnant by a known donor, or if your ex is an asshole whom you wouldn't trust with a dog and he is willing to sign away his paternal rights, you need to get this in writing. If you got pregnant by donor insemination and the procedure was overseen by a physician, the doctor generally will take care of the paperwork, but whoever deals with it, your agreement with the other biological parent should state that he has no claim to parentage, custody, or visitation, and your child has no claim to receive child support from him. (For this you will need to swear that you have sufficient income to raise the child alone.)

If your baby's father has already skipped town, you also should see a lawyer to find out how long you have to wait before you can have your local court terminate his parental rights.

Lesbian and Gay Coparenting

Laws and attitudes about gay and lesbian families are in a confusing state of flux. Judging by recent trends, however, gay and lesbian parents may soon have the mixed blessing of being governed by the same laws as heterosexual parents. In the meantime, it's extremely important that you both have a clear understanding of what you expect from each other, how you want to live after your baby is born, and what the attitudes are toward queer families in the state or jurisdiction where your case (when and if there is one) would be heard. You can check with an attorney referred by the Lavender Families Resource Network in Seattle at (206) 325-2643 to find out up-to-date and local information that may be vital in protecting your family.

Domestic Violence

If you're in an abusive relationship, please call a women's shelter, get out of the relationship, and get legal advice. If you are not sure whether you are experiencing domestic violence or not, a shelter also can help you sort out what's going on. I know it can be really hard to leave a batterer, but your legal position (not to mention the physical and emotional well-being of you and your baby) gets worse the longer you stay. According to the American Psychological Association's presidential task force on violence and the family, abusive men are twice as likely to seek custody of their children as nonabusive men. To make matters worse, these guys are awarded custody about as often as the women.

Again, I'm not a lawyer, but I have, as they say, been around the block, and the block is not pretty. So here are some ideas to kick around if you're not married. First, if you think you can get your ex to sign away his parental rights, go for it. This probably will mean that your child will not be entitled to child support, but it's a good arrangement because your kid can still see her father, but any contact will be on your terms. If getting his signature on anything is a pipe dream, some moms have had luck by not telling their batterer they are pregnant, cutting off all contact, and putting someone else's name on the birth certificate (like a famous dead person). Other moms simply disappear without a trace. One creative mom I know quickly dumped the asshole and eloped with a male friend she really trusted. The baby was born after they tied the knot, and guess what—her friend/husband had automatic paternity rights. And in some states a husband's paternity *cannot* be disproved even with a 99.8 percent certain blood test.

The bottom line: Get out and get to a women's shelter or other safe place as soon as possible. Get legal advice, and don't play fair with your former batterer. He lost the privilege of being treated nicely the day he beat you up (if not before). Courts often don't care about domestic violence if the abuse was never directed toward the child, but keep a diary of all abusive contact you have had with him—when he hit you, what he said, and so on. This journal may not be conclusive evidence, but if the record is detailed, it may help to convince a judge that you are not exaggerating your fears.

This was Family Law 101. For more exciting and in-depth information (or to read about what might happen if you procrastinate getting legal advice until it's too late), check out Chapter 11.

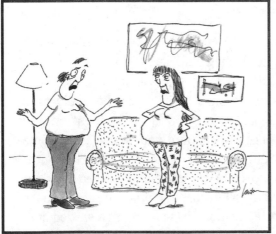

"How can you say I can't relate to your pregnancy?!"

Rebel Mom

Is Marriage Unhip? Not.

Allison Abner, writer mom, author of Finding Our Way

Did you and your partner plan your pregnancy?

Well, I always thought I would have a baby in my late twenties, but when I hit my late twenties it was getting scarier and scarier for me. I wasn't really a baby person—the idea of taking care of a completely needy and dependent person—I could only think of it in the abstract. I was with somebody who really wanted to get married and really wanted to have a baby. We finally made the decision that we really did want to have a baby, we set the date so I could finish my book first (*Finding Our Way: The Teen Girl's Survival Guide*), but then we sort of jumped the gun.

And all of a sudden you were pregnant?

Yes. And then it was very real, and the question for me now was *What am I going to do?* This was it. This was a crossroads for me. Which path was I going to walk down? If I didn't have this baby, I was going to have to break up with him, because it would be over. Or was I going to accept my feelings for him? Was he The One? I was looking at this person with this caption under his head, you know, "The One."

Scary.

I was feeling dizzy, I was almost blacking out. I was kind of in shock.

Did you ever feel like there was a conflict between being a feminist and having this traditional family?

The problem that I had always had with feminism, and I am a very strong feminist, is that among certain groups of people, women have been made to feel like they have to choose between marriage and feminism. Marriage doesn't compromise your feminism; it's whom you pick to marry that could compromise it.

**If your fairy godmama had appeared then, what
would you have asked?**

I would have wanted to know *What are the advantages and disadvantages of getting married because you are having a baby?*

And what would she have told you?

Make a list of the pros and cons. For me, it has helped to deepen the
commitment. But there are pros and cons. Obviously they're different for everyone, but the number-one con is that it's very hard to get
out of. It's very painful and very sticky (and very expensive).
Marriage is a legal agreement, so we went to see a lawyer to find out
more. In terms of the baby's rights and our rights as parents, it
seemed better to be married.

Did you make the right decision?

Yeah. I think I did. I never imagined having a baby by myself. It
would just be too scary to think about doing it all by myself. I had
always seen it as a shared responsibility. You don't have to be married to have that kind of partnership. It doesn't take the marriage
thing. It just takes a commitment.

What about the career thing?

How to deal with her career ambitions is a choice every mom makes.
Do you curb your ambitions, or do you just change them? Because
what you are doing with a baby is juggling time. Maybe you temper
your ambition, or maybe you go in a different direction. I don't feel
like I lost anything by becoming a mother. Having a baby makes you
focus on what's important and what your values are. I think it takes
people who don't have kids—and people who don't slow their lives
down when they do have kids—longer to get to that place. What's
ironic is that now I'm doing what I always wanted to do. I'm staying
home and writing. Having a baby forced me to figure out how to do
that. It forced me to focus on building the life I always wanted.

There is so much to think about and do while we are pregnant, life
can start to seem like a nine-month-long to-do list, but my best
advice remains this: Whenever you can, and as often as you can, crawl
into bed with a magazine or a journal and relax. You'll need the
energy for labor.

Chapter 2
Childbirth Sucks

Natural childbirth? What a time to give up drugs.
—*Lily Tomlin*

"Sure, childbirth is a beautiful experience," says Karen, a twenty-eight-year-old mom who read all about natural childbirth before she went into labor. "As long as it's happening to someone else." Karen laughs when she remembers the night she went into labor. "I was like, whoa, who's the freak who said this wouldn't hurt if I just breathed right?"

She and her coach-husband followed their Lamaze training to a T and managed ("just barely") to get through her labor drug-free, but having read that childbirth didn't have to be painful, Karen was almost embarrassed to tell friends how heinous it was.

Of course, not everyone will tell you that labor can be pain-free, but you're likely to hear exaggerations in one direction or the other.

At seventeen, Elaine was psyched to have her first child naturally and had heard good things about the alternative birth center at her local hospital. All she needed was her doctor's signature, and she could start preparing for a natural birth in a "homelike setting." She didn't have any choice when it came to obstetricians—there was one guy in town who accepted her government medical insurance—so she was at his mercy.

"You don't want natural childbirth," her oh-so-enlightened doctor growled. "You ever watched football? You seen it when those guys get injured? You seen it when they're all busted up and their limbs are broken and their bones are popping out of their skin? Having a baby hurts a hundred times more than that."

Elaine took her permission slip and slouched away, defeated.

If any doctor ever says this to you, please take a picture of him, affix it to this small poster, make a hundred copies, and post it all over town.

It took a couple of days and some encouragement from her aunt before Elaine went back to her asshole-doctor's office to make a scene. He finally signed the form, and just before midnight on July 4, she had her baby girl naturally, with fireworks exploding outside her birth center window.

See, it's not that childbirth is all mystical and painless and beautiful. Childbirth sucks. And this is precisely why you don't need any barking doctor who uses sports metaphors to torture you while you're giving birth, or anyone to tell you that good women don't scream.

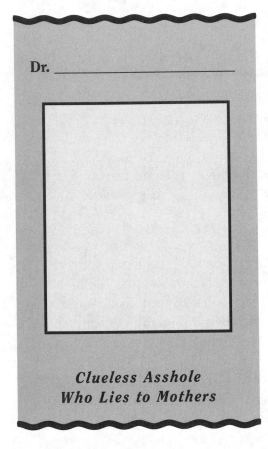

Dr. _____

*Clueless Asshole
Who Lies to Mothers*

I happen to be down with the natural childbirth movement, but there are plenty of women I know and like who think epidural pain relief rivals only the washing machine in terms of awesome inventions. Rosie O'Donnell adopted her child and said, "I got the epidural anyway."

Whichever way you decide to go, however, you need to learn about *both* natural childbirth *and* all the drugs and interventions that can be used during labor. Chances are, things will go as planned, but for every woman who changes her mind or experiences complications that lead to medical intervention during labor, there's another whose epidural doesn't take.

Your Basic Rules of Childbirth

- Choose where you want to be when giving birth.

- Make comprehensive labor and delivery plans in advance and have your birth partner(s) help you stick to them except in an absolute emergency.

- Write your plan down. Make sure everyone has a copy (See "Your Birth Plan," page 58)

- You (and nature) are allowed to change your minds—have a "plan B" you can live with.

- If you're modest, get over it. Lots of people are going to see your crotch . . . and more.

- Don't panic. You can get yourself pretty damn worked up, and it doesn't help matters much.

- In addition to your partner, have a doula, midwife, and/or a friend who has given birth on call to come to your labor. You can always kick people out who are annoying you, but it would suck to end up alone with a doctor and a couple of drug-happy nurses.

- Know your rights, know your rights, know your rights.

- Refuse to agree to any intervention you are not comfortable with and threaten to sue if your wishes are being ignored.

- Feel free to rage at your partner and later deny any memory of the event.

- If you're going to the hospital, don't take public transportation. Call a cab.

Childbirth Denial

"**I** always thought before I was pregnant that I would want a midwife instead of a doctor, but now I feel like I don't want to make a big deal out of this birth," my friend Juana told me a few weeks into her second trimester. She'd just survived the pain and uncertainty of the amniocentesis and the other tests her doctor had performed because she was an "older" mom. "I don't want someone coming into my life and telling me what to do."

I could understand the sentiment. What if a purer-than-thou matron suddenly waltzed into your doing-the-best-I-can life and wouldn't let you have an epidural, or looked down her nose with scorn when you popped open the occasional Diet Coke? It could get very annoying. But the truth is, most midwives are cooler than this pro-medical establishment society we live in has taught us to believe. As I talked to Juana about this, she began to describe the competent but cold obstetrician at her hospital. I, in turn, told the stories I knew of traumatic births and easy births, midwives who supported women giving birth and midwives who panicked. She started reconsidering.

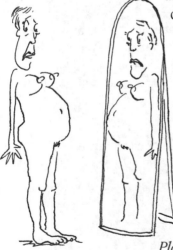

She smiled when I told her that not wanting to make a big deal about birth was like not wanting to make a big deal out of nuclear war.

"Yeah," she said. "I think I'm in childbirth denial."

Of course I was exaggerating—a little—about the nuclear war thing, but birth can be a serious bummer when you wind up with an insensitive practitioner or in a bureaucratic hospital. It's not that I think everyone absolutely *has* to have a midwife, but I think it's important to make an informed birth plan.

Sheila Kitzinger's book *Your Baby, Your Way: Making Pregnancy Decisions and Birth Plans* is a good resource when you are getting down to the details. Talk to midwives, doulas, childbirth assistants, and friends who have had babies. Find out what the options are in your area, and see which helpers and which birth places feel right. Your insurance may limit your choice of hospitals, or your lack of insurance may veer you toward a cheaper—and just as safe—home birth. A birth center is often a good alternative, as it can offer "the best of both worlds" in terms of a comfortable setting, medical technologies on hand in case you need them, and a full-time clean-up staff.

When it comes to helpers, it's cool to have at least one supportive person besides your partner and your midwife to help you out. The best person is a close friend who has had children herself, but you can find a professional by asking moms you know for recommendations, calling the American College of Nurse-Midwives at (888) 643-9433, or checking your phone book under midwives and/or birth centers. If you are giving birth at home you'll probably want two midwives, or a midwife and a doula—one to focus on the baby's needs and one to focus on *your* well-being. In a hospital or birth center, you'll have to follow their policies, but you may be able to have the obstetricians as backup and a midwife to give you her undivided attention and keep you informed of your options each step of the way.

Once you find a practitioner, if not before, you will probably enroll in some kind of childbirth preparedness class where they can go over all the gory details with you and your birth partner. These classes will generally include natural birth techniques from one or more well-known theorists.

Lamaze stresses breathing exercises and concentrating on a focal point to keep your mind off the pain. The Lamaze method (or Lamaze-Pavlov) spurred the natural childbirth movement of the 1960s and inspired countless sitcom directors to have their mothers-to-be imitate panting dogs on prime-time television.

Read, or the Dick-Read method, was developed in the 1930s and stresses different breathing exercises for the various stages of labor as well as a claim that much of the pain of labor was due to the "fear tension pain syndrome." While Dick has a point, we also have him to thank for the idea that, if it hurts, we just aren't highly evolved enough.

LeBoyer is famous for his underwater births. But in or out of water, he's all for "birth without violence," and his method stresses gentle delivery in a relaxing, quiet, dimly lit room with minimum interference. To foster the mama-baby bond, LeBoyer recognized that the newborn should be placed on mom's abdomen and massaged immediately after birth, then gently washed in warm water.

Bradley focuses on a husband coach and encourages the continuation of normal activities through the first stage of labor. The Bradley method is often referred to as husband-coached childbirth and seems to be somewhat responsible for all those guys you see at the hospital wearing sweats, baseball caps, and stopwatches around their necks as they wander the halls murmuring something about the bottom of the ninth inning.

Ina May Gaskin is the legendary radical-hippie-home-birth-guru whose followers are quoted in her 1977 book, *Spiritual Midwifery*, saying things like "I realized that if I loosened up, the pain would go away and everything would be psychedelic and Holy." Considered the goddess of modern direct-entry midwifery, her work is largely responsible for the rise in home births and back-to-nature approach to childbirth of the past few decades. Call The Farm in Summertown, Tennessee, to get her books and videos. (See "Survival Notes.")

What It Costs*

Home birth attended by a midwife, including pre- and postnatal care	$800–$1,500
Pre- and postnatal care and attendance at hospital birth by a midwife	about $1,000 plus hospital fees
Vaginal birth attended by an obstetrician and certified nurse midwife in a hospital	about $2,500
Cesarean birth in a hospital and postnatal care after surgery	about $5,000
Fancy 4-star-hotel-type "birthing center suite"	$7,000
Attendance at birth by a professional doula	about $300–$600

*Talk to your insurance company about what they will cover.

I t is hoped that, along the way, you'll also learn to relax on demand and trust your body. You'll get that baby out, one way or another.

Who Are These People?

Direct-Entry Midwife: A direct-entry, or lay, midwife generally has not been to nursing or medical school but has studied and attended births as an apprentice and studied the prenatal, labor, birth, and postnatal process extensively. While direct-entry midwives are allowed to practice in only a few states, most are at least as competent as folks who have been to medical school. They respect the fact that birth is not an illness but a whole-body experience that has the potential to be majorly traumatic or majorly transformative.

Doula: A doula is a woman whose job it is to support you emotionally, help you with childbirth preparation, and provide continuous support throughout your labor and delivery. You need to find a doula whom you trust and feel comfortable with, but it is also a good idea to find one who has some experience working in the hospital or other setting where you will be delivering. There are also doulas who specialize in postpartum care. Call (800) 45-DOULA for a referral.

Certified Labor Assistant: Certified labor assistants focus on mom's empowerment and well-being during the birth process. You can get a referral by calling the Association of Labor Assistants at (617) 441-2500.

Certified Nurse-Midwife: A CNM is a registered nurse with special training in advising pregnant women and assisting during labor and delivery. According to the American College of Nurse-Midwives, about 85 percent of CNMs work in hospitals or birthing centers and about 4 percent of CNM-attended births are home births.

Obstetrician: An obstetrician is a person who's been to medical school and specialized in pregnancy and childbirth, so she'll know what to do if something goes medically wrong. She may or may not treat childbirth as a natural process and may or may not respect your birth plan wishes. It is extremely important to interview your potential OB to make sure she shares your view of labor and childbirth.

Birth Coach: While the child's father, your husband, or your partner usually ends up with this job, single moms should find a friend (preferably one who has given birth) to fill in. Birth coaches, or birth partners, should go to childbirth classes with you and be there throughout your labor and delivery.

Anesthesiologist: It is an anesthesiologist's job to knock you out. You may not have much choice about who this character is, but ask your primary midwife or obstetrician to tell you all about your birth place's policies on this.

Home Birth

Having your baby at home can seem scary if you don't know many people who have done it, but many moms find their initial worries transform into total enthusiasm for the idea when they start to read and learn about the safety of delivering at home. About 1 percent of births in the United States—30,000 a year—take place at home these days, and moms choose it for all kinds of reasons.

Home birth is cheaper than hospital delivery, parents can remain in charge of the birth process, and without unfamiliar hospital staff running in and out of your room, the experience can be much more intimate and private. Interventions and epidural pain relief also become, essentially, out of the question.

You will need a backup plan for hospital transfer if something goes wrong, but emergency transfers are very rare. This is partly because home birth practitioners will approve only low-risk pregnancies.

While birth is never risk-free, there are no studies showing that hospital births are safer. A 1976 Stanford University study, for example, compared over 1,000 home and 1,000 hospital births and found no significant differences in maternal or infant mortality. A 1992 *American Journal of Public Health* study comparing lay-midwife-attended home births and physician-attended hospital births found home birth just as safe too. As my friend Justine says, "When I tell people I had both my kids at home, they always call me brave, but I think they're the brave ones—giving up all the control to a hospital staff."

Home birth is legal in all fifty states, but some states limit the types of practitioners they will license, and not all birth facilitators are insured for home births.

If you want to have your baby at home, you will have to take the initiative in planning and finding the right practitioners. And don't expect much support from the medical community. You are up against a culture and medical establishment that thinks of maternity as an illness rather than a natural process.

You can call the American College of Nurse Midwives at (888) 643-9433 to get a referral for a CNM in your area. Ina May Gaskin, the revolutionary midwife, also has all kinds of resources waiting for mamas at The Farm in Summertown, Tennessee. They publish *The Birth Gazette* and have videos, audios, and books on birth. Give them a call at (615) 964-3798. The Farm's clinic also offers referrals to home-birth practitioners around the country. They're at (615) 964-2293.

"I had Benjamin at the hospital, and I had a really hard time with the doctors, but I could tell that this was something I could have easily done in my own bedroom," my friend Carrie says. "So when I got pregnant again, we decided to stay away from the maternity ward altogether. It actually turned out to be easier than the hospital birth. I didn't have to worry about what the doctors were going to do, because they weren't there. I had two great midwives I trusted, and Dana was born just fine."

Important Things to Ponder When You Are a Week Past Your Due Date and Still Waiting

- Could this have been a psychosomatic pregnancy all along?
- Has a woman ever been pregnant for, say, a year? Five?
- Do babies pick their parents, or do we live in an anarchist, chaotic universe?
- Is this, perhaps, not the right astrological sign for my child to be born under? Could she be waiting for the next one?
- Will I ever fit into my old clothes?
- Is there life on Mars?
- If there is life on Mars, how long is an alien's gestation?
- Would you have to push harder if you were birthing without gravity?

How Your Labor Might Go

Let me begin with a disclaimer: I have no idea how your labor will go. The first contraction might hit you like a ton of bricks, or you might ease into the process with the grace of a dancer. Your labor may take a few intense hours, or you may be cursing me and my antidrug bias for two weeks. Every woman's labor is different, and while there is a lot you can do to ensure that your process goes the way you envision it, the Hindus were right when they attributed birth to Kali, the goddess of chaos. Just when I think I have a clear picture of a "normal" labor and delivery, I talk to a mom whose experience blows my mind. Having said that, here's a little road map of Kali country—or how your labor *might* go:

Early Labor: Pizza, Beer, and Orgasms

We all know how labor begins—we've seen it on TV and in the movies a hundred times. Mom looks like she's got a basketball under her shirt, and she's walking around minding her own business when all of a sudden—wham!—she falls back onto the couch and looks like she's been attacked by a panther. This sends her partner and more than a few strangers into slapstick panic and convulsions. After speeding through blizzards, crashing a few cars, and dealing with a taxi driver who doesn't speak English, mom gets to the hospital just in time to contort her face under fluorescent lights and give birth. Hell, there are no stages of labor at all. The whole thing can be wrapped up in less than half an hour, and it's entertaining to boot.

Please put all of these Hollywood images of labor out of your mind immediately. Your baby is not going to be born in the back of the Camaro you hitch a ride to the hospital in. In real life, you are a lot more likely to get to the hospital too early rather than too late. Granted, a baby was recently born on BART, the subway system in the San Francisco Bay area, but he was the first and probably the last.

In early labor, you should be able to go on with normal activities, including sleep. My friend Julie went into labor during a three-hour midterm. She finished the test (and got an A), went home and slept for a few hours, and didn't call me to watch her other kids until about 2 A.M.

You Know You're About to Go into Labor When . . .

- your cervix starts to dilate and the little mucus plug that has been protecting the opening to your uterus falls out looking like a big pink-tinged spit wad in your underwear (gross, but true). This could happen days or hours before active labor.

- a steady trickle or gush of liquid comes out of your vagina. ("I'm peeing and I can't stop!") This means that your "water," or amniotic sac, has broken. If you are not already in active labor when this happens, you'll want to call your midwife and head over to the hospital or birthing center. (Some folks recommend carrying around a jar of pickles at the end of your pregnancy—if you're in a public place when your water breaks you can drop the pickle jar and, perhaps, avoid some embarrassment . . . but whatever.)

- you feel like someone has slipped you some acid, you've been on your hands and knees cleaning a heater vent with a Q-tip for two days, or strangers start running up to you in the town square screaming "Get home! Do you want to have that baby in the piazza?"

- you start having contractions—which feel like nasty and intense menstrual cramps or a tightening and hardening sensation—they last about forty seconds and may or may not come at regular intervals. Early contractions can go on for hours or days before you actually need to go to the hospital, but give your midwife a call if you think it's time or when your contractions are coming regularly five minutes apart—whichever comes first.

If you don't have a midterm, however, you should spend your early labor walking, taking showers (providing your water hasn't broken and someone is home to help you out), having sex if your water hasn't broken, and gently celebrating. As one nurse suggests in *Our Bodies, Ourselves*: Eat pizza, drink a beer, and have orgasms. You can probably do without the beer, but these things can help you relax and stimulate contractions. During this mostly tolerable stage of labor, your uterine and cervical muscles are expanding and contracting to stretch your cervix—the neck of the womb—to its limit of about 10 centimeters.

While you don't have to rush off to the hospital, do call your midwife or doctor whenever you think "This Is It." She can help you decide when to do what. There are a couple of different theories about when you should get to the hospital or birth center, and they depend almost entirely on how cool the place you plan to give birth is. Maternity wards and birthing centers can be okay places to hang out for the long hours of early labor, and many moms feel more comfortable knowing that they don't have to drive across town. Some maternity wards, however, are no fun at all. And home, if it's not too messy, can be a nicer place to spend the day or night. In any case, by the time your contractions are coming regularly five minutes apart, call someone.

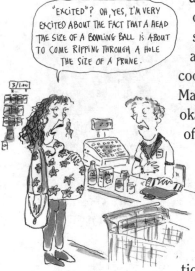

"EXCITED"? OH, YES, I'M VERY EXCITED ABOUT THE FACT THAT A HEAD THE SIZE OF A BOWLING BALL IS ABOUT TO COME RIPPING THROUGH A HOLE THE SIZE OF A PRUNE.

Transition: Suicide, Homicide, and Despair

Just when you're almost completely dilated and you're beginning to think childbirth might not be so terrible after all, "transition" hits. It's that last centimeter that's the bitch. Time stands still for what seems like a long, long time. You may, like my friend Kamara, threaten to kill a few people—frightened husband included. You may, like Dionne, attempt to jump out the hospital window. Your legs might tremble and cramp, you might puke, and you'll probably want to push before you are quite ready.

When I was in labor, I still believed the popular myth that when it was all over, a "strange amnesia" would set in and I would forget the pain. I never did forget, but fearing that amnesia, I scrawled a panicked note to myself during transition: "NEVER DO THIS AGAIN."

What can I tell you about this time of despair except that it won't last forever? It must have been women in labor who popularized the proverb "The darkest hour is just before dawn."

In *The American Way of Birth*, Jessica Mitford wrote that she was reassured to discover "the word 'travel' is derived from 'travail,' denoting the pains of childbirth. There is in truth a similarity between the two conditions." And she was right. The only other time I had scrawled those four words, I was on a thirty-six-hour bus trip down a half-paved Tibetan highway: "NEVER DO THIS AGAIN."

I usually hate it when people say things like "no pain, no gain," or "such and such makes it all worthwhile," but the birth of a tiny new soul or a long-awaited arrival in Lhasa are about as magical as it gets. Exhaustion suddenly feels like enlightenment, and pain—although never forgotten—takes on the quality of a mystical and provocative initiation.

Scream!

Screaming during labor and childbirth may be considered taboo in more than a few cultures, American included. All the more reason to do it. You don't want to get yourself worked into a panic, but if you're prone to modesty, consider this: You are lying/sitting/squatting/standing there butt naked and sweating with your legs open and no matter how poised you are, you've got a really unflattering look on your face. It's time to throw modesty to the wind.

The Final Frontier: Exhaustion, Relief, and Elation

I hesitate to tell you much about the end of labor—when you will at last push your baby out and meet her face-to-face—because there is little chance you will remember any of my words.

When, finally, your cervix has dilated enough for the baby to come out, your doctor or midwife will give you the go ahead. "Push." It's best not to be lying on your back to push the baby out—squatting, kneeling, or lying on your side are the best positions to help your baby out. But as one loser obstetrician told my friend just as she was lying naturally on her side about to give birth, "I don't deliver on the side."

Kind of like "I don't do windows." But whether you are "allowed" to deliver the way your body tells you is right, or if someone else makes that decision, know that many millions of babies have gotten out—of women smaller than you or I, no doubt.

If you have epidural pain relief, it will have to be turned down so that you can feel your body enough to push. "Many women feel torn between bearing down with all their might to get the baby out and holding back, afraid that the head is going to rip right through them" according to the Body Shop authors of *Mamatoto*. But you have to push, and you have to push *hard*. This is a magical time, but it's also a scary time, and your helpers may even get a little panicky. You may end up pushing for twenty minutes or two hours before you feel a burning sensation, and the baby's head crowns and he is then tugged, or he slides, out into the world.

Everything will happen quickly then—your suddenly empty belly will tremble; your baby will take his first breath; some more pushing and you'll get the placenta out; your partner, midwife, or doctor will deal with the umbilical cord; and you will see and touch your child for the first time.

What can I tell you? Whether you are horrified or elated, breathe these moments in. Amnesia won't take them away from you.

What's the Deal with Medical Intervention?

Despite the natural childbirth movement, many hospitals still routinely employ a twisted little cycle of unnecessary intervention that can actually complicate your labor, rather than help things along. Many interventions require electronic fetal monitoring, which, in turn, requires that you lie still, and lying still is pretty much guaranteed to make your contractions less effective and more painful leading to—you guessed it—more intervention. Not surprisingly, low-income moms and women who go into labor without a doula or midwife advocate are most vulnerable to hospital policies that are motivated by pressure from insurance companies, fear of malpractice suits, and general misogyny.

When I had my daughter, the goddess smiled on me and gave me a relatively quick (ten-hour) and uncomplicated labor. But because the nurses and doctors at the hospital where I was giving birth had just gotten a bunch of new gadgets they wanted to try out, I was subjected to a fair amount of torture.

The Italian hospital staff left me alone through most of my early labor, and I did a good job scaring them away during transition by cursing in English when they tried to come near me with their needles. They laughed and called my boyfriend and me "the Gypsies from the North." But just when I'd had enough of the natural hell of labor and I was crouched in the corner of the bathroom plotting my own suicide and several murders—my little hospital gown and out-of-control hair making me the picture-perfect lobotomy candidate—one of the nurses found me and, apparently sensing my vulnerability, started screaming at me in Italian. As I stood up, my water broke and the nurse shoved me into a wheelchair and pushed me into the dreaded delivery room. There the torture crew lifted me out of the wheelchair, dropped me onto a metal table, clamped my ankles into restraints, and started chanting *"spingere."*

My sister and my baby's dad, who had gotten into the room somehow, screamed "no drugs" and held back a blond nurse with a giant needle in her hand. Meanwhile, apparently because I was not pushing hard enough, a second nurse held my jaw shut while a third produced a wide leather strap from beneath the table and pulled it down tight over my belly in a bizarre attempt to push the baby out herself. While I tried to push and keep track of all the insanity, a guy I'd never seen before (my OB was on vacation) stared between my legs and then, shouting something, suddenly sliced into my perineum. As he was reaching for the forceps he wouldn't need, my daughter popped out. A split second later, a nurse threw all the doctor's tools into a deep metal sink and they crashed, metal on metal, welcoming my daughter to this harsh, harsh world.

Fortunately for you, much of this drama is rare. (I have never heard of another victim of the leather strap, for example.) And fortunately for me and my daughter, Maia, none of this seems to have caused us lasting damage. But, being young and trusting and kind of lame, I never even *asked* about these things beforehand.

Medical intervention is unnecessary in a normal labor, so the obvious moral here is to find out if your practitioner uses any routine procedures, and keep in mind that you have the right to refuse intervention. If complications do arise, you'll probably welcome any tricks your doctor or midwife has up her sleeve, but even then, it is important that your practitioner explains—each step of the way—what is being done and why.

Here's a list of the most common procedures and when they are appropriate. I deleted "prepping" (or shaving your pubic hair) from my original list because it has become all but obsolete in the past couple of years, so if your doctor suggests this, make sure you tell him he's obsolete.

Intervention	Why It's Cool	Why It Sucks
Epidural (painkillers injected in your spine area)	Self-explanatory: *Painkillers.* If you've made an informed decision and/or if you end up having a long and traumatic labor, go for it.	May not "take," may make it difficult for you to push, requires fetal monitoring, requires you to stay still, may lead to further intervention such as drugs to speed up second-stage labor and/ or pushing phase.
Enemas (pumping water in your butt so you'll have diarrhea)	May make you feel better and may prevent you from pooping during delivery (as if you'll care at that point).	Totally unnecessary, may make you feel *worse,* which may make you request an epidural.
Electronic fetal monitoring (external and internal)	If you have an epidural anesthesia, induced or accelerated labor, it becomes necessary.	It's never been proven safe, it may be uncomfortable, and it requires that you lie down.
Lying down	It's not. But it's required if you've got a fetal monitor going.	Increases risk of fetal distress, slows or stops productive labor, leads to further intervention to speed labor back up.

Rupturing the amniotic sac (popping your water)	Can speed up your labor and make contractions more effective if done after you are 4 to 5 cm dilated and totally effaced; may allow your practitioner to better check for fetal distress after you're about 8 cm dilated.	Some doctors will rupture the membrane in early labor just to speed things up. If you ask me, doctors who do this routinely need to take some 'ludes themselves and leave your labor (and your water) alone.
IV	In rare cases when you are puking everything you drink, an IV can help keep you hydrated.	Many hospitals give every woman in labor an IV "just in case." IVs make it difficult for you to move around and, in normal labors, are totally unnecessary.
Pitocin (a drug used to induce or accelerate labor)	If there's a question about the baby's survival, if you have toxemia or maternal diabetes, an induced or accelerated labor may be a good alternative to a C-section.	Your baby has to be constantly monitored, an intensified labor means more pain, it may lead to further intervention, and it's often used for convenience rather than out of necessity.
Episiotomy (a cut through skin and muscles between the vagina and anus to enlarge opening)	It's not, although some say it decreases your chance of tearing. You have the right to refuse episiotomy.	Midwifery techniques (perineal massage and/ or applying hot compresses or warm oil for relaxation) can minimize tearing, so the cut is unnecessary; may damage sexual sensation later; and stitches may be painful.

Vacuum extraction and forceps (used to pull the baby out)	If you are unable to push hard enough (because you've had an epidural, for example), if the cord is around the baby's neck, or if there's fetal distress, may be a good alternative to a C-section.	Unless the baby is having trouble getting out, vacuum extraction and forceps are totally unnecessary and may hurt your baby's head.
Cesarean section	The goal with childbirth is to get the baby out. C-sections save lives, and (if you'll excuse my shallow vanity) the scar will hardly be noticeable once it heals.	Beware of practitioners and hospitals with C-section rates over about 15 percent. Many have rates of less than 5 percent. The surgery is overused and takes a good six weeks to recover from.

Your Birth Plan

A birth plan is simply a list of your preferences and requests with a little introductory paragraph that says something like "I want to have clear explanations of all medical procedures, of my progress, and of any complications that arise. I agree to accept medical judgments and interventions with my informed consent only if there is a medical emergency for either me or my baby. I would like the following requests honored," or "I wish to have an epidural as soon as possible and I agree to accept other medical judgments and interventions with my and/or my birth partner's informed consent. I would like the following preferences honored . . ."

Think about the following options. You may want to have them on your request list:

❑ Do not use electronic fetal monitoring—internal or external—unless there is fetal distress.

❑ Do not use an IV unless it is an emergency.

❑ I want to have more than one support person.

❑ I do not want to be separated from my birth partner during my hospital stay.

❑ I do not want an enema.

❑ Do not shave my pubic hair.

❑ I want epidural pain relief.

❑ I do not want epidural pain relief or any drugs during labor.

❑ I want to be allowed to walk and move around during labor.

❑ I want to be allowed to wear my own clothes during labor.

❑ I do not want the amniotic sac artificially ruptured.

❑ I do not want Pitocin to induce labor.

❑ I want my birth partner to be allowed to cut the cord after it stops pulsing unless it was wrapped around the baby's neck.

❑ If a cesarean becomes necessary, I want my birth partner to accompany me in the operating and recovery rooms.

❑ I do not want any bright lights.

❑ I would like to deliver in any position I choose.

❑ I would like to deliver in a quiet room.

❑ I do not want an episiotomy; we'll use perineal massage instead.

❑ Immediately place baby on my belly for nursing after birth.

❑ The baby is not to be removed from my sight.

❑ Allow forty-five minutes for delivery of placenta.

❑ I plan to breast-feed. Do not introduce anything artificial to the baby.

❑ I want to be discharged from the hospital as soon as possible after birth.

❑ If hospital stay becomes necessary because of complications, I wish to have the baby in my room with me.

When you talk to your midwife, obstetrician, and other moms, you may want to add other concerns to your list. Don't worry about too many requests, but keep them clear and to the point. It is hoped that your doctor and everyone at the hospital or birthing center where you've chosen to give birth will be cool and on your side, but making a birth plan can also help you think clearly about your wishes.

And Remember . . .

- Childbirth is a natural process, not an illness.

- Having a baby always hurts.

- Doctors may be more worried about a malpractice suit than about your health or your baby's health.

- Unnecessary fetal monitoring will prolong your labor because it requires you to be lying still. You need to walk around to keep your labor progressing.

- The "need to push" that childbirth educators are always talking about feels an awful lot like the need to poop.

- You have the right to give birth without medical intervention.

- If medical intervention becomes necessary, it's not your fault, and you have not "missed out."

- If a guy tells you that his wife was only in labor for two hours with her first child, he means that he was only awake for two of the hours.

The Best-Laid Plans: Dealing with Disappointments

"I did not have a beautiful home birth," says Janelle. "I know that there are a lot of unnecessary C-sections, but mine was a case where a C-section would have been the best thing."

"It was really grueling," Stephanie tells me as she's recovering from an unexpected cesarean. "And disappointing."

Often when things don't go as planned in labor, we are left feeling that we have somehow missed out, we wonder what we could have done differently, and we blame ourselves for not being somehow better. As my friend Delma tells me about her C-section, "I felt as if I'd failed as a woman."

Please put these notions out of your head. Many, many great women have had C-sections. Thoughts like these are signs of classic mother guilt, and whether your labor goes well or complications arise, you need to remember this: You did the best you could with the information you had. And this: Your birth experience was, simply, your birth experience. No two labors or deliveries are going to be alike, so please don't feel like yours was "wrong." As your child grows up, she will ask about her birth, and believe me, if things didn't go as planned, your story will be all the more exciting.

Although Janelle waited five years to write about her home birth and her son's subsequent stay in the Intensive Care Unit, she told friends the whole story almost immediately. We need to tell people. We need to write about what happened. We need to allow ourselves to grieve the disappointments.

Life is weird. And then you're stronger.

About Circumcision

Circumcision is the surgical removal of the foreskin, a loose piece of skin that covers the head of the penis. Although long performed by Jews and Muslims for religious reasons, IT IS NOT MEDICALLY NECESSARY. Still, about a million babies in the United States (about half of all newborn boys) are circumcised each year. The surgery, which costs about $250 and lasts fifteen minutes, is extremely painful, and is usually done without anesthesia, a tradition left over from the old school belief that newborns do not feel pain. While some people claim that the circumcised penis is easier to keep clean, the operation can create at least as many problems as it prevents. If you are thinking about getting your boy circumcised, please consider your decision very carefully. As Betty Katz-Sperich, an anti-circumcision nurse and activist, says, "It's [also] a Jewish tradition to be very thoughtful and not just do things without thinking about them."

And with the steady decline in routine circumcision over the past few decades, your uncircumcised son will be far from "alone" in the locker room.

If you are of two minds about the procedure, viewing *The Nurses of St. Vincent: Saying "No" to Circumcision* (available for $29 from

Fireball Films, P.O. Box 107, New York, NY 10003), will definitely convince you (or, perhaps, the partner you've been trying to sway) not to do it. In the short documentary, six nurses tell what they saw in the circumcision room that led them to inform the doctors at the New Mexico hospital where they worked that they would no longer help with the procedure. The video also includes chilling close-up footage of an infant circumcision. Call me a lightweight, but I could hardly *watch* it, let alone imagine putting my kid through it.

Call the National Center for Education in Child and Maternal Health at (202) 625-8400 or National Organization of Circumcision Information Resource Centers at (415) 454-5669 for more information.

If you do decide to leave your son's penis alone, watch out for old-school doctors who do not know how to care for the uncircumcised penis. Often they will recommend all manner of scrubbing and cleaning and pulling back of the foreskin. All of this scrubbing can actually cause the infections you are trying to prevent. As with every part of a new baby, you want to be gentle with the penis. Use warm water and keep your baby clean, but know that the foreskin is a natural thing and the penis is, essentially, a self-cleaning little appliance.

Name Calling

"I can't tell you how many names I tried on when I was pregnant," Xan says. "I don't know why, but the name meant everything to me. I could call her Sunflower and move out to the country and feed her only organics. Or I could call him Malcolm and teach him to be a strong black man. Or I could call the baby Lee and never worry about sex discrimination."

As Xan knows, the real reason pregnancy takes nine months is so that you have time to come up with a really cool name. You have time to roll it around on your tongue. To say it softly in the shower. To get really into Greek mythology and consider "Zeus" before your friends laugh at you and make you veto it. You have time to find out what the names you've always liked mean. You have time to think about old family names and names that represent your baby's heritage.

In Mormon, Gypsy, and other traditions, babies are given a secret name in addition to their first names. Among some Gypsies, this secret name is whispered to the newborn and never spoken again until the child reaches puberty. It is intended to deceive demons who, not knowing the child's real identity, will have no power over it.

These days, choosing a last name can take almost as much consideration as choosing a first name. Sure, for some people it's obvious. The traditional thing to do is to name the baby after dad. But if you're a single mom, for example, you may want to lay a matrilineal claim right off the bat. Hyphenated names, I hear, are losing popularity as those of us who grew up hyphenated in the '70s become parents. But when the names sound good together, it's certainly worth thinking about.

Some families I know are deciding to toss out their last names all together in favor of brand-new ones. I know a mom whose last name is BraveWoman. I always assumed she was born with the name, until I met her son, Mr. BraveMan.

My daughter's last name is Swift, which is totally made up—her dad originally introduced himself to me as Mr. Swift, so by the time he fessed up to being a "Smith," I was already attached to the original. Don't ask. Anyway, if you can't think of a name, don't panic. That's how people end up getting called things like "Crisis." (Yes, it's happened.) Something will come to you.

My sister was one of those people who had boy and girl names picked out when we were, like, ten, but when she got pregnant, nothing sounded quite right. Then she went into labor at Leonardo da Vinci airport in Rome and, voilà, I had a nephew named Leonardo. Another mom I know just looked through the list of babies recently born at the hospital where she was in labor with her son. "Julian" sounded cute, so she snagged the name.

I know a guy named Christian whose mother picked up the birth certificate, looked at the blank after "First or Christian Name," and circled "Christian." He's just lucky she didn't circle "First."

And when I was born, my mother was so tripped out by the fact that I was a girl and she hadn't thought up any femme names, she ended up waiting until I was three months old to call me anything at all. My birth certificate says "Gore Girl," and I have a "Supplementary Name Certificate" with the "Ariel Fiona" part filled in. Actually, I've never seen the name certificate, so for all I know my official name is really "Girl." But, honestly, wouldn't you rather be called "baby" for three months than walk around for a hundred years answering to "Oscar"?

Below is a subjective list of fifty very cool names, but as long as I can persuade you not to name your child after a beverage, I'll consider my role as an author successful. At this point I've met a Cappuccino, a Daiquiri, a Chardonnay Chablis, a Water, and an Ice. Maybe it's just me, but naming a baby after a drink just doesn't seem nice.

FIFTY VERY COOL NAMES

A Subjective List (or Where My Hippie Heart Is Revealed)

Aaron	Indigo	Raven
Aisha	Jaden or Jade	Sam
Ali	Jake or Giacomo	Saskia
Anais	Jasper	Saul
Angel	Jeremiah	Selena
Chiara	Lillianne	Shena
Dakota	Luca	Sinclair
Danica	Madison	Sylvan
Eva	Maia or Maya	Taisha
Ezekiel	Malcolm	Theo
Farai	Marcos	Tillie
Francisco or	Max	Trevor
Frances	Meeko	Xan or Alexandria
Freya	Miles	Zachary
Hannah	Natalia	Zenobia
Harper	Nicholas	Zolton
Hunter	Pablo	Zora

~~~~~~~~~~~~~~~

Rebel Mom

Getting Your Way

Julie Bowles, family advocate and mama of three

You've attended a lot of hospital births with low-income moms. What kind of care do they tend to get?

If you are just poor, but you don't look poor in a stereotypical sense, then you get treated all right. But if you are very young, or of color, or if you don't speak English, then the hospital staff tends to want to make all the decisions for you, even if you've made a birth plan. Often the nurse will offer only a partial explanation for why she is doing an intervention, and she may minimize what the consequences of the intervention will be. This is true even if the mother has an advocate with her.

Do you think these problems only affect poor women, or are all moms at risk?

I think all moms are at risk, especially if you haven't done a lot of research in picking a birth attendant. It comes down to rights. A lot of doctors, especially those on the white, male side of things, think they have the right to make decisions for you and tell you what to do. Poor women are at particular risk because, especially if you've been poor all your life, you haven't had a lot of practice demanding quality, and labor is a very hard time to start.

What can we do before we go into labor to avoid being mistreated?

We can make sure we know about our bodies and the process of birth, we can pick a birth attendant who respects us, and we should take along two advocates. We should also know what the mortality statistics are—not many babies die because of lack of intervention. Most of us would be just fine without any doctors at all. C-sections are really only necessary in a small percentage of births, but some hospitals run as high as 34 percent. Of course, if you want painkillers, then you can certainly have them. And if a C-section is necessary, then of course you should have one. The problems come when they are giving you things you don't want, and when they are not fully explaining why they are doing things.

How about once we're in labor, say we end up at the hospital without our midwife or partner?

Try to remember what your original goals were, try to remember the facts about intervention, and keep in mind that the hospital staff may not always be giving you the whole story. Of course, not all hospitals and doctors are going to mistreat you, but it's common enough for me to feel this strongly about it. One of the reasons you want to have more than one advocate is so that you won't end up at the hospital alone. You also need to remember that "no" means "no." If you don't want a certain intervention, threaten to sue them if they won't listen to you. The other thing to remember is that you are paying to have these people treat you the way they are treating you, and even if it's not coming directly out of your pocket, someone is paying for it, and nobody wants to pay for you to be mistreated.

Some people say that you shouldn't go around making scenes because you might offend someone who will later be called on to save your life. What's up with that theory?

The bottom line is that they have to save your life even if you have offended them. That's what the Hippocratic Oath is all about. And if you are ever going to make a scene, labor would be the time to do it.

Let's say we do the best we can to prepare for childbirth, and we do the best we can while we're in labor, but shit still doesn't go the way we wanted it to.

Even if you don't remember to do all those things I mentioned before, you still did what came naturally to you, and that is okay. You should write nasty letters to whomever you think deserves them, talk to lots of cool moms, drink tea, relax, and enjoy your new baby. After the fact, the important thing is to come into acceptance of whatever happened.

A few days after I had Maia, my sister came over to our apartment and commented that she felt like there was something only women who had children knew, something we couldn't let her in on even if we wanted to. "You know," she said, "it's like that sense you get from recovered heroin addicts or that bond you notice between thieves, like they've been somewhere and seen something that you're not even sure you want to know about . . ." And then she left me sitting on my couch, nursing my newborn, and pondering this strange analogy: Junkies. Thieves. And Mothers. *Hmmm . . .*

Several years later I learned that in old religions they say that after childbirth, mothers remain for some time in the underworld. We have been and we have seen, and it takes a while to get back aboveground. Maybe that's what my sister was talking about.

Chapter 3

Hey, Baby

It feels like I'm baby-sitting in the Twilight Zone.
*I keep waiting for the parents to show up because
we are out of chips and Diet Cokes.*
—*Anne Lamott,* Operating Instructions

"All of a sudden I had this little creature who looked like an alien," remembers Michelle, a twenty-year-old single mom. "I was full of all these crazy emotions, I felt like Courtney Love and a Hallmark card all mushed into one."

Michelle left the hospital with her daughter the day she was born and had help from her own mother and friends when she got home, but by nightfall it was just Michelle and the newborn in their quiet apartment. "I tried to sleep, and the baby woke up a few times, but *I* woke up every fifteen minutes, just to look at her," she remembers. "You know, when you're in a foreign country, and you dream and you wake up thinking you're at home, and then you look around in the dark and remember where you are? That's what it was like."

Few moments in life are as emotional and amazing and soul-shattering as the first hours and days after a baby is born. But we all (well, most of us) manage to pull through. There's nothing like the smell of a milky newborn in your arms as you're curled up in your favorite chair, and there's nothing quite like the wails that come in the middle of the night, just as you've finally fallen asleep. You feel like a victim of one those evil sleep-deprivation experiments and, if you're like me, you start having some startlingly violent thoughts.

Some women describe the first few days after a baby's birth as euphoric, but after about day three, most of us experience some form of postpartum blues, ranging from a little tearfulness and exhaustion to seriously psychotic episodes. Not only are we hormonally challenged, but all of a sudden we're not pregnant, *we're moms*. Our bodies are completely out of whack, our emotions are all over the place, and we're not getting any damn sleep. A chemist might disagree with me, but the closest comparison I can come up with is this: Electric Kool-Aid Acid Test.

"Did you ever think you could love anyone so much?" a friend asked me when we got home from the hospital. And I shook my head, sincerely overcome with tenderness for this new life. So it was all the more frightening when, later that day, I sat at another friend's house staring into the fire and rocking the baby back and forth, desperate to make her stop crying—and for a split second I honestly felt like throwing that baby right into the flames. What stopped me wasn't my unconditional love and instinct to protect my daughter, even from myself. What stopped me was this thought, which flashed in my mind like a revelation: "I do not want Jo Beth Williams to play me in a miniseries." And neither do you. I scooted my chair back away from the fire and stood up, holding Maia close to my chest. She was still crying as I scurried into the kitchen and handed her to my friend. "I'll make the pasta," I said. "Just deal with her."

It's understandable that we're not going to love being a mom all the time. Still, it was several years before I found out that my momentary psychosis was actually pretty normal. The important thing is that we don't act on these bizarre impulses. If you do think you are going to really lose it, or if depression lasts for more than a couple of days, you should talk to a professional. Your best bet is to find someone with experience in postpartum depression or to start with a confidential hot line. Otherwise, talk to friends and other moms you know, and when you feel your grip on reality and your new motherhood loosening, be good to yourself. It can help to write or review the story of your baby's birth with a friend to process both the joyful moments of childbirth as well as your disappointments. Relax, get as much help as you can, sleep when the baby sleeps, eat well, and drink a lot of water. And give yourself a break when you need one.

Culture Shock

I hate to keep harping on the negative here, but as Anne Lamott says, "Having a baby is like getting the world's worst roommate. Like Janis Joplin with a bad hangover and PMS." And anyway, you probably won't need much help getting through the blissful times when the baby sleeps all morning, wakes up for a half hour to nurse, and then passes out again, sweetly gurgling.

It's those *other* times. Those times when your childless yuppie chowderhead friend pops in with a darling gift and your house is trashed and the baby is spitting up all over the place and you look like a cross between Bon Jovi and Frankenstein; those times when you haven't had adult human contact in what feels like a lifetime even if it's only been eight hours; those times when colic hits and you miss being pregnant and you start to realize how your own mom got to be so weird. It's all those times that seem to come together within a few days or weeks just to burst all your picture-perfect motherhood fantasies.

As Jennifer said when her son was three weeks old, "Does this job have paid vacation or anything?" Unfortunately, it doesn't. But somehow, things are going to get, well, not exactly easier, but more doable. The culture shock will wear off, you'll settle into this new land of motherhood, and, eventually, *you'll* be the experienced mama offering a compassionate smile to new recruits when you see them running harried through the market or half collapsed at the bus stop.

When Maia was about a week old and I was nearly dead from sleep deprivation, I put her in her buggy and made my way up a little hill to our neighborhood café where friends cooed at the baby and offered beer and cappuccino to this newly lactating mom. An acquaintance noticed the dark circles under my eyes, patted my back lightly, and assured me: "The first three months are the hardest. Once you get through that . . ." He paused for a moment, like he was trying to remember what, exactly, would save me after this postnatal trimester. "Once you get through that, you know you can do anything."

I appreciated his brief affirmation that *it wasn't just me*. And, in retrospect, he was right. Lots of folks will tell you that whatever "stage" your kid is in is "the hardest." The first three months extends to the first year, then they tell you your kid is so advanced, he's reached the "terrible twos" ten months early. When everything doesn't turn magically peachy at three, they tell you to wait, "This transition is the hardest." But the guy at the café knew what he was talking about. It's the same advice we give new residents of the San Francisco Bay area after they've felt their first temblor—it's not that the quakes become more predictable, or that they register any lower on the Richter scale, but you do get used to them. You learn to sleep through the mild ones; you bolt your furniture to the walls; you come to expect the aftershocks; and you survive. It's still scary when the earth starts to shift, but you get more confident, and pretty soon you can't imagine living anywhere but right here, at the epicenter. It's just like being a mom.

How Crazed Are You?

At the risk of getting totally yelled at by my psychologist friend when she reads this over for the mental health sensitivity factor, I offer you Quiz #2: How Crazed Are You?

1. Glancing over this quiz, you want to:
   a. answer all the questions because you are bored (the baby sleeps so damn much!).
   b. engage in a little depression derby competition and call another new-mama friend to quiz her about how crazed she is.
   c. slash the pages out of the book and call another new-mama friend to tell her what a bitch she is.

2. When the baby cries in the middle of the night, you:
   a. roll over, whisper "What's up, sweetie?" and gently move the baby from his bassinet to your side so he can nurse.
   b. hit your partner over the head with the baby intercom and say, "Deal with her, you little deep-sleeping shit."

c. start having sick and twisted thoughts about your kid, start crank calling the baby's father and leaving obscene messages, and/or consider faking a case of multiple sclerosis so that Dr. Kevorkian will help you commit suicide.

3. When your friend calls and tells you she's going to Tower, you demand that she pick you up some good:

   a. Mozart and reggae.

   b. Liz Phair and blues.

   c. Nirvana and Hole.

4. When you do lie down to rest, you are sometimes overcome by:

   a. tears and exhaustion.

   b. nightmares, anxiety attacks, and/or feeling like you've lost yourself.

   c. memory loss, paranoia, and strange voices telling you to do bizarre and/or violent things.

5. If they made a miniseries about your first month postpartum, the person(s) who could play you best would be:

   a. Jill from *Home Improvement*.

   b. Roseanne.

   c. Jo Beth Williams and Susan Lucci—playing your dual personalities in alternating scenes.

6. A pint of Ben and Jerry's ice cream sounds:

   a. yummy.

   b. kind of heavy.

   c. blah. "And don't talk about food anymore or I'm going to puke."

7. What you really feel like doing right now is

   a. taking a warm bath, getting a good night's sleep, and waking up at a decent hour to admire your offspring.

   b. running fast and far.

   c. going out and screaming at everyone you meet "I just had a baby, okay?" before you punch them in the stomach.

8. You want to go back to work:
   a. in a while, a long while if possible.
   b. right away even though you don't have a job, just to get you out of the damn house.
   c. never. "I'm totally incompetent and will never be able to get out of bed again, let alone work or talk to anyone."

9. Of all the videos you rent, the one you want to watch again and again is
   a. *Groundhog Day*.
   b. *Basic Instinct*.
   c. *Faster Pussycat, Kill Kill*.

10. When you reexamine your view of yourself as a mom, you decide you are
    a. born to do this.
    b. good enough.
    c. not really a mom. This is all some kind of sick nightmare conspiracy, perhaps orchestrated by a strange international alliance that includes your obstetrician, midwife, partner, and Saddam Hussein.

Scoring: Give yourself 1 point for every A, 2 points for every B, and 4 points for every C.

10 points: June Cleaver. You go. You probably *were* born to this, but try to mess up your hair a little if you want to make other new-mama friends. You're just the kind of chick us harried moms loathe.

11–20 points: Erma Bombeck. You're gonna be fine. Make sure to get help from family and friends and consider joining a support group. Rent a couple of videos from the comedy section and eat popcorn with some friends.

21–30 points: Roseanne. Drink some herbal tea with a few jasmine flowers, call a baby-sitter, and go out to play video games with some cool friends, then get a massage on your way to the shrink. You're probably gonna be okay.

31–40 points: Mommie Dearest. Run, don't walk, and get experienced professional help immediately. I'm serious. Take care of yourself, girlfriend.

Kicking Back

"There's this new store in town that delivers pizza and videos," says Eva, a thirty-five-year-old mother of a newborn. "Pizza *and* videos," she repeats, as if she has just found the promised land. This mama knows that the early days of motherhood are for kicking back with the baby, taking deep breaths, and acting like a queen on her throne. The ideal postpartum survival kit, according to Eva, is a mushroom pizza, chamomile and alfalfa tea, a trashy video, and some good reading material. We're not talking *War and Peace* here, of course. Something more along the lines of *People* magazine will do nicely. A videotape series of the complete *Melrose Place* might even be cool.

If you're much too wholesome for B-movies, you might replace the videos with meditation and the pizza with brown rice and vegetables. If reading and watching TV seems to take too much effort, I think those inspirational/ relaxing/ healing New Age books on tape are pretty awesome. You can call Sounds True Audio at (800) 333-9185 and have them send you something by Clarissa Pinkola Estés, or a nice monk, to kick back with.

Getting Help

In many parts of the world, postpartum care is all but guaranteed—extended family, home health care providers, and other members of the community naturally come over to help you care for yourself and your new baby, prepare food, and keep your house from getting too messy. In India, women are traditionally pampered for the first twenty-two days after their child is born. In Holland, postpartum care is generally taken care of by midwives-in-training who live-in for about a week and a half. I realize it's a little late for you to move halfway around the world, but you might want to casually mention these traditions to anyone who calls and asks how you're doing.

Many moms report getting all the help they need from the well-wishers who come by to catch a glimpse of the newest member of the family. Others have felt totally isolated, because they don't know many people in the area, because the visitors stop coming after a few days, because their partners go back to work very soon, or because they live in the middle of nowhere. If you don't feel like you are getting all the help you need, it's important to let the friends you do have know. Often people stay away because they want to leave you in peace, and they are secretly dying for you to call them up for a favor. Don't worry about being a pain in people's butts. If they don't know how to say "no," that's their problem. And how often do you have a kid, anyway?

Obviously, depending on your life situation, all of this may be really easy or really difficult. I once got a call from a woman I didn't know who had seen my zine. She was using the phone at a homeless shelter on the East Coast where she had just moved, and she told me she was planning to give her baby up to a foster home until she got on her feet. She had found this last-resort practical help, but she needed someone to talk to. I imagine that mine was not the first number she dialed, but she caught me home and I listened to her for a good two hours. I don't know how helpful I was to her in the end, but I do know that when a woman is willing to go out on a limb like that, to call a stranger three thousand miles away on the off chance that the stranger will be cool, she's got what it takes to survive, even in the toughest of circumstances.

Robin Lim, author of *After the Baby's Birth . . . A Woman's Way to Wellness*, suggests tacking a little note to your door that reads: "Glad you are thinking of us. Baby and mom are resting peacefully. We sure would love a helping hand with _____ (housework, errands, the kids, meals, etc.)." This, by the way, is also nicer than putting a sign on your door that reads "GO AWAY." If it doesn't work, you might leave a similar message on friends' and acquaintances' answering machines.

Finally—and this is really cool—there are professional doulas who care for postpartum women and their families. Even if you didn't have a doula attend your birth, you can hire one now. Call your doctor, midwife or (800) 45-DOULA for a referral. The doulas services should run you about $10 to $12 an hour and will be well worth the investment.

Honestly, girls, this is no time to try and be all stoic and self-reliant and I-can-handle-it. There are really only two kinds of new moms: those who get the help they need and those who have nervous breakdowns.

Important Questions to Ponder in Your Spare Time

- Who is the disposable diaper guru who decided the tape should go in the back?
- Do boys and girls really pee all that differently, or are pink and blue diapers just some ad wizard's idea of a joke?
- Is this bathwater really "lukewarm," or have I completely lost my sense of temperature after squirting a dozen different liquids on myself?
- If you're not really supposed to put baby powder on a baby, then what's it for?
- Was my baby Elvis in a past life, or just some peasant?
- If he *was* Elvis, shouldn't I contact some kind of Elvis Lives fan club or something?
- Should I stick one of those ridiculous bows on my daughter's head so that people will stop calling her buster?
- Must the umbilical cord look that weird?
- How much would it cost to get little cards printed up that say "Take a 'lude and get a life," so I wouldn't even have to talk to those losers on the bus who spout useless criticisms of my parenting skills?
- Where does the time go . . . or does it exist at all?

You Can Nurse, Even After Nipple-Piercing

Breast-feeding is totally and absolutely where it's at. Yes, mamas, this is what your tits are for. Well, one of the things. If you're an adoptive mom or if you've had breast surgery in which they cut your milk ducts, you may still be able to get into parts of the nursing thing with your practitioner's help. There are even contraptions that can get formula from a bottle to your baby's mouth via a little tube by your nipple, so babies who can't get breast milk can get the same bonding action as their nursing buddies.

If you are not sure why I'm so into breast-feeding, let me sing its praises for a moment.

- Breast milk is a baby's natural food.
- You won't have to worry about buying formula or anything else for a good four to six months.
- Nursing helps you lose a helluva lot of weight.
- It helps your uterus contract to its original size (no small feat, eh?).
- Breast-feeding helps with bonding.
- Breast milk, and especially the colostrum that comes in before the actual breast milk, is full of antibodies, so you pass your immunity to illnesses down to your babe.
- Breast-fed babies get far fewer ear infections.
- Once you and your kid get the hang of it, nursing is easy and fun.
- You can get free friends at your local La Leche League meeting if you're a nursing mom.
- You won't have to get up in the middle of the night to prepare a bottle. (You'll barely even have to wake up after a few week's practice.)
- If you work or have to be away from your baby, you can pump breast milk into a bottle for feeding.
- Breast-feeding costs less than buying formula.
- And last but not least, it feels good.

As Cathy, a thirty-year-old nursing mom told me, "I live to breast-feed, especially in public."

When word got around in one midwestern town that a woman was being hassled for nursing in a mall (indecent exposure, you know), the local mamas got together and staged a nurse-in. Most fabulous.

If you still think that breast-feeding is not right for you, or if my enthusiasm is just pissing you off because you cannot breast-feed for one reason or another, you have my permission to skip on to the birth control section (as if you need my permission). But if I've sold you on the idea, or, if like about half the moms in the United States, you were already sold before I offered you my humble opinion, I have to tell you that nursing is a learned art. Your midwife, doula, or nurse should help you get started. (This often consists of a stranger nurse grabbing your tit and saying, "Like this.") You can call La Leche League at (800) LA-LECHE for more help. As Timera says, "Natural, my butt. We are not born with any innate ability to nurse. Don't ask me how the first people ever figured it out." In the meantime I offer you these tips gathered from mothers and the Bureau of Maternal and Child Health.

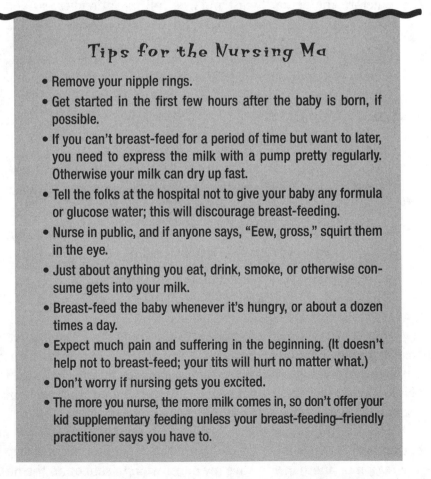

Tips for the Nursing Ma

- Remove your nipple rings.
- Get started in the first few hours after the baby is born, if possible.
- If you can't breast-feed for a period of time but want to later, you need to express the milk with a pump pretty regularly. Otherwise your milk can dry up fast.
- Tell the folks at the hospital not to give your baby any formula or glucose water; this will discourage breast-feeding.
- Nurse in public, and if anyone says, "Eew, gross," squirt them in the eye.
- Just about anything you eat, drink, smoke, or otherwise consume gets into your milk.
- Breast-feed the baby whenever it's hungry, or about a dozen times a day.
- Expect much pain and suffering in the beginning. (It doesn't help not to breast-feed; your tits will hurt no matter what.)
- Don't worry if nursing gets you excited.
- The more you nurse, the more milk comes in, so don't offer your kid supplementary feeding unless your breast-feeding–friendly practitioner says you have to.

- Try to nurse in comfortable spots. Sitting in a big comfy chair with a footrest and a pillow is nice.
- Expect to leak. (You can get nursing pads to soak the booby juice up when you're in public.)
- Always nurse for about the same amount of time on each side—ten to twenty minutes. Burp your babe halfway through and again when your baby is finished eating.

I also must offer you a warning here. We all know that tobacco companies are evil little swines when it comes to marketing cigarettes, but formula companies can be pretty sneaky themselves. They pay hospitals to give you free formula hoping that you'll think these are somehow doctor-endorsed, and they send you coupons for free formula and sweet-looking congratulations for months after you give birth. Then, just when your milk has dried up, it stops being free, and it keeps being less healthy. They may even tell you that supplementary formula feeding will help you in some way. Lies, lies, lies. So here's the Hip Mama General's Warning: Any supplementary formula feeding can be hazardous to your breast-feeding efforts. If you have decided to breast-feed, formula companies are not your friend.

Music to Nurse Your Baby By—Twenty Tried and True Artists and Albums

1. Joan Armatrading, *Track Record* or *Whatever's for Us*
2. *Boys on the Side* soundtrack
3. Tracy Chapman, *New Beginning*
4. John Coltrane, *A Love Supreme*
5. Indigo Girls, *Swamp Ophelia*
6. *Janis Joplin's Greatest Hits*
7. Annie Lennox, *Medusa*
8. Bob Marley, *Legend*
9. Sanjay Mishra with Jerry Garcia, *Blue Incantation*
10. Joni Mitchell
11. *Mozart for Your Mind*
12. Bonnie Rait, *Luck of the Draw*
13. Sade, *Stronger than Pride*
14. Michelle Shocked, *Kind Hearted Woman*
15. Sinéad O'Connor, *Universal Mother*
16. Steel Pulse
17. Sweet Honey in the Rock, *Sacred Ground* or *Still on This Journey*
18. Talking Heads
19. TLC, *CrazySexyCool*
20. *Waiting to Exhale* soundtrack

Mother Earth or Mother Sanity: The Diaper Debate

Around the time Maia was born there was this serious campaign to get moms to stop using disposable diapers. (Does Earth Day 1990 ring a bell?) "You *are* going to get a diaper service, *aren't you?*" everyone wanted to know as soon as I arrived back in California with my infant. "Disposable diapers are just *awful*. They stay in the landfills *forever*."

The environmentalists are right. Cloth is better. Cloth diapering also happens to be cheaper and better for your baby's skin. But don't you think it's just a wee bit fishy that when we all decided we had to save the world, the first people expected to give up their conveniences were us moms?

I used cloth diapers for about six months. I even washed and boiled them myself without a service for three of those months. But eventually I just couldn't take it anymore. What do you do if you're out all day? Carry around plastic bags full of shit, that's what you do. What do you do if the diaper service flakes on you one week? You sit around with a hamper full of shit—as if it weren't already getting seriously nasty after the first seven days. And what happens as your infant matures and starts doing the big, stinky, way-far-from-cute shits? You get shat on, that's what.

I tried the kind of disposable diapers they said were environmentally friendly, but they didn't work, and eventually they took those particular diapers off the market because it turned out they weren't so environmentally friendly after all. Those of you who can go cloth the whole route have my unwavering respect, but when it became a question of my sanity or some shit covered in plastic in a landfill forever—call me a polluter—my sanity won out.

I mean, couldn't we start saving the world somewhere else? Couldn't we ban cars or something? How about just shutting down McDonald's and Exxon? Yes, I have to agree with Erma Bombeck on this one: "I'd rather do away with foam cups and have hot coffee poured into both of my hands and drink fast than do away with disposable diapers."

To Immunize or Not to Immunize?

Within the first six months of your baby's life you will be faced with the decision: to immunize or not to immunize? Actually, information on immunizations will probably not be presented to you as a "decision." Your pediatrician will simply give you a shot schedule as if you have no choice in the matter. But as a parent, you have the right to make medical decisions for your child. The vast majority of babies in the United States are immunized against polio, tetanus, whooping cough, diphtheria, measles, and mumps. But there is a growing movement among parents not to immunize their children.

Some parents do not immunize because they cannot afford to. Others choose not to immunize because they are suspicious of the medical establishment or worried about the side effects of vaccinations.

Most of the controversy focuses on immunizing children in the first few months of life and immunizing them against non–life-threatening illnesses like chicken pox. One safe "compromise" might be to wait until your baby turns one and the natural immunity she got from your breast milk has worn off. Even then, you might want to skip the chicken pox shot.

I had Maia immunized against all the big potentially fatal or crippling illnesses, and would do it again, but the choice is up to you. You can ask your doctor about immunizations, read *The Immunization Decision: A Guide for Parents* by Randall Neustaedter, and get other good information from *Mothering* magazine and the *Birth Gazette*.

Unless You're Ready for Another Babe...

Okay, so you may not be terribly horny for a while, and your baby's probably not going to sleep long enough for anyone to turn you on. But eventually, when you're ready, you are probably going to have sex again.

I'm sure you've heard that you can't get pregnant right after you've had a baby. Maybe you've also heard that nursing is a form of birth control. I'm here to tell you one thing: That's bullshit. If your partner is a man, you can get pregnant. Yes, it's back to those pesky condoms. Until you get refitted for a diaphragm, get the okay from your doctor about the pill (after you've stopped nursing), or started using some other form of birth control, condoms with foam or jelly are your best bet. And remember, condoms don't do any good if they are just sitting on the nightstand.

Party On

Most cool religious traditions include special rituals and celebrations for the birth of a new baby—there are christenings, baptisms, blessing ways, ceremonial rum or beer parties, placenta burying rituals and birth trees, feasts, and all kinds of carryings on, depending on what tradition you're down with. But what if you don't follow any particular religion? Celebrate anyway, of course. Whether you decide to party right away or wait a couple of weeks, a *Welcome to the World* party of some sort is definitely in order. Here are some ideas:

- One of the points of a christening is to bring together the community of friends that your kid will be able to count on throughout life. So, if you're not Christian, you can leave the religious part out and invite all your close friends whom you know your family can count on. Have each person bring an artistic offering—a dance or a song or something, to welcome baby to the planet.

- Have a housecleaning party. (I am so serious.)

- In Jamaica, folks crack open a bottle of rum when there's a new member of the family. Play some Peter Tosh and share drinks with friends.

- Don't lift a finger. Have a Martha Stewart friend organize the whole thing—just tell her what kind of tea cakes you want and watch it all magically appear.

- If you don't have a Martha Stewart friend, make it a potluck.

- If the placenta doesn't gross you out too badly, have a party where you bury it and plant an oak. Otherwise, just plant a birth tree without the afterbirth. (Most hospitals will let you take the placenta home if you request it. Hell, in Berkeley, California, they've been known to give it to mom with a little tree even if she doesn't want it.)

- Get a live band, invite a bunch of friends, sit with your baby in a really comfortable chair, and just hold court like you're the queen of the world. (You are.)

~~~~~~~~~~~~~~~~~~~~~~~~~~~~~~~~

Rebel Dad

Making the Leap from "Guy" to "Dad"

Glen Bergers, aspiring artist, founding member of the
garage band Family Values, and endless retail slug

Did you attend the birth of your son?

Yes, we had Jasper at home. We had two midwives attend the birth—
they worked together and had delivered about 800 babies, that's
more than a lot of doctors can boast.

**Was it difficult to figure out how you fit into this
new family when it was your wife who gave birth
and breast-fed and everything?**

I was a very active participant. A lot of the first year is just holding
the baby and getting the baby to eat and getting the baby to sleep.
We shared that, but Tina [his mother] was more important to Jasper
at that point. Part of the reason we made the decision to have the
home birth was so that we could experience it together as much as
possible.

Tina and I met at a pretty wild time in my life, and we were kind of
friends for about a year. Then things sparked up. We conceived
Jasper the second time we ever made love, so it happened pretty
quickly. When she called to let me know, I just knew right away that
it was okay. I wasn't even really thinking toward the future.

**So, you didn't really have an established relation-
ship before you knew you would be parents?**

Nine months plus probably two months. It was sudden, but I never
really felt shock at the time. In retrospect, I feel like I should have
freaked out. Maybe I just felt like I knew what the future would be
like. There were no guarantees at all, I guess you could throw the
word "lucky" in there. It's not always easy or happy, but most of the
time it is. The greatest challenge of being a family is being able to
balance and arrange the business of being a family, how you are
going to have enough money.

Did division of labor become an issue for you guys?

It's been different issues at different times. Until Jasper was five, I was the only person who worked. We wanted Jasper to have an extended bonding period [with Tina]. He breast-fed until he was almost four. That bothered a lot of people, even people with kids, but I didn't see anything wrong with it. I always saw what Tina did with Jasper and at home as a job, so it wasn't an issue for me that I was the one working outside the home. You learn everything as you go along. Sometimes you learn from making a mistake, and sometimes you learn from just doing the right thing the first time.

Do you have any advice for other men on how they can make the transition from guy to dad more gracefully?

I don't know. I think that the relationship Tina and I entered into was as much a potential mistake as it was a success. It was kind of lucky, it was kind of accidental, but being a dad was also a part of me. I didn't have any big plans at that time. I guess I would say, just take being a dad seriously.

After Jasper was born, I found great inspiration and warmth in being a father.

There's a real energy to expecting a baby. I don't know if a lot of men experience it in the same way I did. I know men who are very distant about it, but I cut Jasper's umbilical cord. Tina practically choked me when she was giving birth. I got really into it. I got slimy. I knew at that time that this was going to have life-changing potential. Maybe it was because our relationship was very new—we were so impassioned and excited. I don't know if I ever stopped to ask myself about the future. Maybe that's a good thing, not to ask those questions, not to worry about it. Jobs and money can change, but you've got to get all the emotions in place, and the love.

Once we get all those emotions in place; once we come back "down to earth" after the exciting, crazy-making, depressing, magical journey to motherhood; once we survive those first, tentative months and get used to living at the epicenter, it's time to take a deep breath. Motherhood is a radicalizing experience. And your personal mama revolution has only just begun.

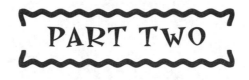

PART TWO

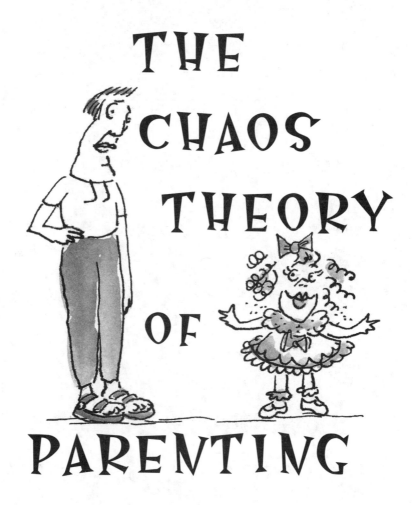

THE CHAOS THEORY OF PARENTING

Chapter 4

Toddler Avengers

I always wanted my kids to question authority, just not mine.
                                                    —Eve, fifty-four

As I turn down the cereal isle at the supermarket to grab a box of Cheerios, I see a puffy-haired and blushing young woman standing over a screaming toddler who looks like he's break-dancing on the hard tile floor. At least five people near the cereal boxes stand freeze-frame staring toward the mother and child.

After a moment's pause I pick up a family-size box of toasted O's, hand it to Maia who is perched in the front of our shopping cart, and push past the scene, whispering "Watch your head" to the baby and "It happens to the best of us" to the woman, who smiles, even though she looks as if she is about to die of embarrassment. Turning into the dairy section, I pause in front of a yogurt display to thank the goddess of tantrums that, at least today, it wasn't my kid.

Walking, talking, testing new limits, weaning, potty-training, separation anxiety, temper tantrums: Welcome to toddlerhood, ain't it beautiful?

The Screaming Mad Hullabaloo

You know it's your worst nightmare: a toddler temper tantrum in *public*. We get dreadfully embarrassed, we are at least as frustrated as our kid, and we've got *shit to do* in the bank or at the grocery store or wherever we are when it hits. "Those lights in those places make kids crazy," says the old folk singer Utah Philips. "We all know that."

Shopping cart accidents alone send some 25,000 kids to the emergency room every year, and every mom who's ever been to the store knows how all these injuries happen—the little rebels are screaming and flailing about, grabbing for this treat and that brightly colored goodie, and they're driving us absolutely batty. But what can we do?

If we can't leave them at home with someone (c'mon, since when did banking and grocery shopping count as "quality time"), then we have to wing it. We can shop at smaller stores, preferably where they don't have those lights. We can offer our kids healthy treats when they're in the cart (who cares if the checkout guy gives you a dirty look?); we can prepare emotionally to be interrupted. And finally we can surrender. We may not be able to grab that loaf of bread they keep obnoxiously hidden in a back corner of the store, we may get bizarre parenting advice screamed or whispered at us in the frozen-food aisle, but we survive.

"You can just feel everything starting to fall apart," Antol tells me. "Then, within maybe thirty seconds, my son is freaking out completely, and as if everyone else in the store hasn't noticed, they start on the loudspeaker going, 'clean-up on aisle five . . . mayonnaise on aisle six . . . broken glass on aisle seven,' like they're sportscasting for my kid's demolition derby."

You'll probably be both reassured and horrified to hear that these dreaded public outings and the tantrums kids throw at the most inopportune moments cause a whole heck of a lot of child abuse. This is because we, as parents, are totally unsupported in most communities. We are put under this tremendous unspoken pressure to appear to have well-behaved children, to appear to be always happy, to appear to be causing no trouble as we go about our business. Our kids, in turn, not only feel the pressure, but they are either bored out of their gourds in line at the bank, or they are surrounded by marvelous things in the store and they want them all. And then, of course, there are those lights that make us all crazy.

At home, tantrums are always easier to deal with. There are no bright lights we can't dim, there are no stranger's eyes staring at us from behind boxes of cereal, and there are no errands we just have to *get done*. But those high-pitched screams and howls, wherever they let loose, can still be way past annoying.

So what can we do when our kids throw their howling tantrums at home? Honestly? We can encourage them. I am completely serious. Toddlerhood is an extremely frustrating time to live through. That notorious twentysomething angst can't hold a candle to two-year-old angst. Imagine being three feet tall, wanting everything but not having the language to ask for it. Imagine knowing enough about the world to see that your mother's leaving but not quite understanding the concept that she'll be back. Imagine knowing enough about the world to see that the big folks use toilets but try as you might to figure out the whole timing thing, you shit in your pants. Imagine depending on a bunch of grown-ups with their own issues for absolutely everything.

A Few Things to Remember About Public Tantrums If They're Beginning to Get the Better of Ya:

- They aren't anyone's "fault."

- In turn-of-the-millennium fluorescent-lit America, they are basically inevitable.

- It may help to dye your hair green, wear a tattered biker jacket, and walk around muttering "I don't care what you think of my family, you little punks."

- It may help to write a letter to your local newspaper declaring that if some entrepreneur would do your errands for cheap, you'd be his first customer.

- As your kids grow, these uncontrollable outbursts will happen less and less—this is a stage!—I promise.

Granted, being two can be a blast, but even the most nostalgic-for-those-days-without-so-many-responsibilities among us have to admit that toddlerhood can also be hell. So, as long as your kid isn't hurting himself or anyone else, let those emotions rip. You can offer your commentary—"I'm sorry you're feeling so frustrated," "I can see that you're angry with me," even "You are driving me insane, so I need to leave the room until you're ready to do something else"—but there's no reason to make any bigger deal about your kids' negative emotions than you do about their positive ones. Sure, at least one neighbor will knock on your door and either accuse you of child abuse or threaten to call the authorities on you, but you can calmly explain that you believe children have a right to express their emotions. Or, better yet, you can forget to answer the door when you see that loser coming up the walkway with her panties in a wad.

If you still have mixed feelings about this approach, consider the fact that our kids will need to have perfected the temper tantrum if they're ever going to be revolutionaries worth their salt. "She'd be fabulous at a sit-in," Anna says as her daughter goes limp when she tries to move her mid-fit. Let's hope the reflex comes in handy someday.

Before we leave the subject, I have a little secret to tell you about the screaming mad hullabaloo. We often think, as my friend Kimberly puts it, that "my kids are totally out of hand when they're with me, but they're perfect when other people watch them. They must seriously hate me." But actually, it's just the opposite. Most kids act out *either* when they are with us *or* when they are off with a sitter. This isn't always the case with very young children, but as they get older, it's almost universal. Take the eighteen-month-old who plays quietly at preschool all day, and then all of a sudden when mom picks her up, bam! She's wailing. Does the kid hate her mom? Does she want to stay at preschool longer? Is the teacher lying when she claims that the child doesn't do this at school? No, no, and no. On the contrary, Mama. The kid digs you. She feels safe with you. And she's been saving every little one of her pissy emotions all day long just for you. *Great*, you're thinking. *Thanks a lot*. But our kids learn, really early on, that being happy and cute and quiet are the more socially acceptable emotions; while anger, fear, and frustration, whenever possible, need to be saved up and expressed in a safe place.

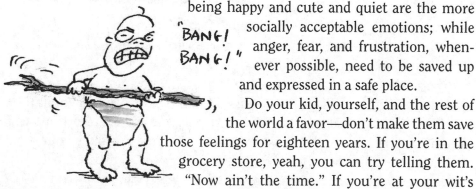

Do your kid, yourself, and the rest of the world a favor—don't make them save those feelings for eighteen years. If you're in the grocery store, yeah, you can try telling them. "Now ain't the time." If you're at your wit's

Fun Ways to Be Largely Ineffectual as a Parent

(or How to Change the Subject and Introduce BIG WORDS)

Problem	Solution
You want to talk to your kid about something she may or may not be in trouble for so you tell her, to "Please come here." She refuses, thus bringing up a possible second offense you have to deal with.	Say "Buddy, I feel a power struggle coming on and I'm already planning to hold my ground." This won't do any good, but it's never too soon to introduce the whole "power struggle" concept.
You are convinced that your child is being "manipulative" and therefore think you should punish him.	Say "I think this is bringing up other issues for me, so I'm going to have to withdraw from the argument." This won't do any good, but it will introduce the concept that moms and dads, unlike gods and goddesses, have their own problems.
Your kid wants to go the farmer's market wearing a Hello Kitty bathing suit, rainboots, and a snow jacket.	Point out that this outfit is, while incredibly hip, incongruous with accepted beliefs about weather. Then offer her a hat and leggings to go with the ensemble.
You put your kid on time-out, setting the timer according to the old *1 minute x age* formula, but the kid won't stay in the dreaded chair.	Repeat the rules about time-out over and over until the buzzer rings. Then offer an extra minute in *lecture* time. This will so annoy them that they'll just sit through the next time-out.

| Your kid is flailing around on the floor, screaming "Bad mama, funky mama, bad mama." | Say "I'm sorry that you are angry at me, but I'm sure glad you are able to express it so eloquently." This won't do any good either, but being ineffectual is average—being ineffectual *and* respectful, well, that's pretty awesome. |

end, you can offer them a cookie to shut them up. But when you can, and as often as you can, give them a safe place to get that shit out of their systems.

Closing the Milk Bar

The worldwide average age for weaning is four. This is partly because food is a scarce commodity in many parts of the world, so as long as you can get the perfect food for free, why waste it?

If you can afford to feed your baby without breast milk, you get to weigh all the other factors in your life and decide when is best for you—and your kid—to close the milk bar. A quick survey of doctors, midwives, and nursing advocates puts the "proper age" for weaning somewhere between eight months and five years. Some people will tell you that six or eight months is far too early, others declare that nursing a five-year-old is obscene, but if you've learned anything as a mom, it's probably that "people" are full of it. Trust your own instincts.

Sometimes children will simply "wean themselves" after as little as eight months or a year, but a child-led weaning often won't happen until around the age of four unless you get pregnant again, start exercising a lot, or do something else that dramatically changes the taste of your milk. The bottom line is that if you don't want to go on nursing throughout your kid's preschool years, you may very well have to put some effort into it. Remember that there's nothing wrong with initiating the weaning process yourself whether it's conflicting with work, your kid has started biting, or you simply want to reclaim your body. The important things are not to stress out too much, not to make your kid feel like you are pushing her away, and not to make her feel bad for wanting to nurse.

I started weaning Maia when she was two, by curtailing her nursing in public. (I admit it—the dirty looks were getting to me.) By the time she was three, she didn't nurse at all except at bedtime, and she finally quit completely when she was four. Of course, it helped that I didn't mind her nursing and that I wasn't working full-time, but even if you choose to close the milk bar sooner than I did, a gradual approach is nice. Babies tend to be hooked on nursing for a few different reasons. First of all, it's food. Beyond their nutritional needs, it tastes good, if you smoke they are probably addicted to the nicotine, and most important, babies come to associate closeness, cuddling, and peace with suckling at your breast.

Tillie, the mother of an eighteen-month-old, had planned to nurse her son until he "weaned himself," but after a year and a half of nursing eight to twelve times a day, she couldn't take it anymore. She started shame spiraling because she felt like she "should" be sticking to her plan and "should" be able to continue giving her son what he wanted. But she knew herself pretty well, so when resentment and anger starting creeping in every time her son asked for "nursey," she knew she had to wean him. It was more important for her to close the milk bar gradually—taking care not to make her son feel like she was pushing him away—than for her to stick to her "Plan A" and wind up having some big end-of-Mama's-rope blow-up.

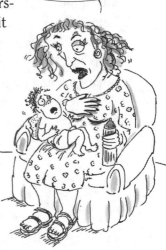

"SORRY, THESE ARE NO LONGER USER FRIENDLY."

Tillie's gradual plan went something like this: First she stopped nursing him in public, then she established a special place in the house "just for nursing." Neither of these things decreased the number of times her son nursed every day, but she was able to introduce the whole "the store will be closing in ten minutes, please bring your purchases to the register" concept. After three months of gradually nursing her son less and less, she just stopped, explaining that she would cuddle him and be there with him, but couldn't nurse him any longer. There were a couple of really hard days, physically painful for both mom and son, but they did it. They had to.

STILL BREASTFEEDING?

BREAK THE HABIT WITH NEW NIPPLETTE® GUM!

I NEVER THOUGHT I'D QUIT...

(NIPPLETTE)

Theresa, the mother of a six-year-old, tells me that her daughter still asks if she can have a little taste. When Theresa told her that her breasts were empty and trying to nurse would be like "trying to drink apple juice out of an empty jug," her daughter laughed, but they got to talking about other things that might be just as comforting. Her daughter dug this word, "comforting," and at first tried to convince Theresa that, perhaps, a new Lego set would do the trick. When her mom didn't fall for it, the little girl agreed that a cup of tea and a back rub would be pretty "comforting."

Obviously, it's harder to negotiate with younger kids, and some of them end up being pretty violently opposed to the idea of closing the milk bar, but baby massages, holding (in positions that don't remind them too much of nursing), and an assurance that they are simply moving on can help tremendously.

If you're having trouble, don't hesitate to call La Leche League and talk to other moms. Weaning can be a hard one. It's been three years since I did it with my daughter, and my tits hurt just thinking about it.

Potty Training

Perhaps you've heard the pop-psych theory of potty training. It goes something like this: Your timing as mom/personal potty trainer is everything. It's not the sun sign or the moon sign your child was born under, not nature or the eighteen-some-odd years of nurturing that you'll put in that will determine your kid's personality, it's when you potty train 'em. According to this theory, the kids who get forced out of diapers too soon turn out, well, anal retentive; the kids who get potty-trained too late turn into major slackers; and, of course, those lucky few toddlers who get taught how to use a toilet right on time turn out just right.

Now, the main problem with this little theory is that it does not include a date, only more pressure for us to "get it right already." I can pretty much guarantee that you'll hear this theory or a similar one attached to the ages eighteen months, two years, two and a half, three, and so on. Somewhere near the end of your kid's career in diapers you'll also hear the occasional "Damn, that baby still wearin' diapers?" or the ever-helpful "I'm sorry, our day care *does* take infants as young as six months, but they really do have to be potty-trained."

This isn't to say that all the pressure to get your kid out of diapers comes from outside—it's nice not to have to change those disgusting diapers anymore; your kid will finally look like she's got a regular butt; and toilet paper really is a good bit cheaper than disposable, or even cloth, diapers. Having said all of this, toilet training isn't anything you must, or should, rush. Timing may be everything, but every kid's inner clock is different, and if you don't make a huge deal out of it, 90 percent of children will potty train themselves—right on time—between the ages of about eighteen months and three years.

One mom describes her last-ditch attempt to get her two-and-a-half-year-old on the toilet: "Finally I just told him, 'Bad!' I was really tired of it all and I just said 'It's bad to go to the bathroom in your pants.' It seemed to work too. He stopped having bowel movements in his pants, so I assumed he was using the toilet. It was, like, three months before the lady at his preschool told me that the minute I left him there every morning, he'd go in his pants. I was standing there listening to this and it suddenly occurred to me that he'd been holding it whenever he was with me—maybe all weekend sometimes—I felt so awful."

One thing to know about potty training, as well as what makes some kids wet their beds throughout their childhoods, is that a great deal of it is genetic. Some children potty train themselves as early as eighteen months, and this really is the earliest age when kids' muscles and nerves are developed enough even to be able to control urination and poops. Before kids can be potty trained, their bladders and bowels have to get big enough to store waste for a period of time. This usually doesn't happen until they are about two and a half. Once you're dealing with children who are physically ready, they also have to have the communication, understanding, and motor skills required for the whole operation. Basically, we're looking at some time between the ages of twenty-eight and forty-two months, and even then, toilet training is a pretty long process. You might want to start by putting a little potty in the bathroom and talking about what it's for. It's natural if all of this tries your patience, but attempt to be mellow. I've made fun of the pop-psych theory, but the truth is that people can end up with a lot of trauma from potty training, either because they were forced to control themselves too soon or because their parents started freaking out about the situation.

One little girl I know just started using the potty by herself when she turned two. Her mom was hesitant, in the beginning, to get the girl her own little toilet because she thought they were "gross," but since her daughter was into doing this thing privately, often not telling her mom until she needed a little help wiping, the little potty helped a lot.

Another mom tells me that she thought her son would "never" get out of diapers. But she sat him on the toilet periodically for about six months and somehow, although he "never seemed to have any interest in actually going to the bathroom while he was sitting there," he finally did get it.

I've heard that some parents put that fish-shape cat food in their kids' potty and then instruct Junior to "sink it." Or they use O-shape cereal and say it's time for target practice. Now, this sounds a little gross to me, but whatever works.

"So, who's your personal potty trainer?"

My daughter was on the older side when I finally got her out of diapers. I waited until the summer after she turned three, when it was warm enough for her to go around in her underwear and I wasn't too busy with work or school. At that point, I just told her I thought it was time and not to worry if it took a while to get used to. She had accidents for a few days (and I let her wear pull-ups to bed), but she got it pretty quickly. If all that means that she'll grow up to be a slacker, well, worse things have happened.

On Rage, Spanking, and the Rest of It

There is something both annoying and interesting that happens to many moms as our kids grow up—we get these weird flashbacks. They generally start when our kids hit the age of our own first memories, if not before, and they continue through the years. Some moms I know report being bothered by remembering—at every turn—what *their* parents would have done; how *they* would have felt as kids. But a great opportunity for empathy comes with the periodic comparisons between our kids and ourselves as kids. Sometimes we gain new empathy for our own parents. More important, we gain new empathy for our kids.

"We don't hit at all," one mom tells me. "But there was definitely some spanking in my house when I was little, and sometimes, when my son is so rude to me, I just want to spank him. My brain just tells me that that's the right thing to do."

The natural thing to do when we become moms is to parent in the same way we were parented. Or, depending on our upbringing, to do everything in our power to be exactly the opposite of our own parents. But it's important to remember—especially in times of stress when we tend to revert to autopilot (or autoparent, as the case may be)—that we do not have to be our mothers and that we do not have to *not* be our mothers. A simple philosophy made when we aren't upset can help. Mine goes something like this: Treat my daughter with respect; remember how the world seemed when I was her size; listen to her point of view before I offer mine; bend rules; never hit; warn her about consequences; follow through; and apologize when I blow it.

I recently met an older friend's son, and although I knew how old he was long before I laid eyes on him, somehow seeing this grown man who was almost twice as big as his mother left me speechless. As we were leaving the bar where we met, I whispered to my friend, "I'm totally traumatized. Is my kid ever going to be that big?"

She nodded. "If physical punishments are your main source of control, eventually you will lose." Of course, the thought of getting totally creamed when our kids hit sixteen isn't the only reason not to hit them, but it's something to keep in mind. You can also get in some serious shit with the authorities if you hit your kid with anything but your open hand. But even that open hand and the nasty, shaming words that hurt the spirit instead of the body cause pain, violate trust, and, honestly, only make the little rebel scream louder.

One time when Maia was about one and a half, she would not stop screaming and throwing my books all over the house. I tried everything: reason, time-out, bribery, empathy, screaming. Finally I'd had enough and I slapped her across her little red, pudgy face. I will never forget the shock and horror in her eyes. But do you know what happened after that heartbreakingly silent pause? She screamed even louder and threw even more books. I never hit my daughter again, but I've heard parents who hit their children on a regular basis say things like "It's the only thing that works." If it really worked, though, you'd only have to do it once, and as every abusive mom discovers, you "have to" do it again and again and again.

There is, of course, a difference between rage, which we don't need to dump on our kids, and anger that we just express and that we don't need any specific response from. You know you're in rightful, in-the-moment anger when your kid draws on the wall and you say, "Hey, we don't draw on the wall," and you clean it up or ask them to clean it up, and then it's over. You can be pretty sure the little doodle on your nice white wall is bringing up other issues for you, however, if you start screaming and running around the house and telling your kid what you're going to do if he ever pulls that shit again.

The French educator Françoise Dolto says, simply, "Teach them what comes from your heart." And the Mexican feminist Anilú Elías adds, "If the rudeness of a child bothers you, don't be permissive, because sooner or later, words will jump out of you that wound the spirit and that you will regret; if it pains you when a child cries from being punished . . . don't act the disciplinarian, for it will break your heart."

Sometimes when I'm starting to feel even crazier than usual, I just sit down and write a letter to someone who has hurt me and another to someone who has been cool. Obviously I don't plan to send these letters anywhere, but we have to dump our baggage somewhere—on paper, on our poor therapists, on politicians, on the people who have really fucked us up—we have to dump our shit where it won't hurt anyone, especially our kids.

If you can't scream and get too crazy because your kids are around, try writing out your rage. It can be kind of scary to allow ourselves to rage, but when we give all our pissy, negative crap a home and let ourselves get really into every little taboo feeling, we actually become less rageful, and we take a few steps toward forgiveness. Folks will tell you that it's not okay to feel like throwing your kids off a bridge and then joining them in the murder suicide, but, if you ask me, it's just not okay to *do* it. And it's not okay to tell your kids about these fleeting urges.

Chill Out

- Take up kickboxing.
- Write a letter in your very private "id book."
- Give your kid a time-out if she needs to cool down, and take one yourself.
- Take a bath and drink some chamomile tea.
- Get a baby-sitter.
- Go to a gym and hit a punching bag.
- Call your local loser politician and scream in his answering machine about his latest pathetic move.
- Call your ex and don't let him/her get a word in edgewise (presuming he/she doesn't already have a restraining order to protect him/her from such outbursts).

- Take a deep breath and say to your kid, "I'm sorry, I'm about to lose my last marble, and I don't want to freak out at you, so excuse me while I go have a psychotic episode in my room."
- Go in the backyard and throw neon paint at your fence.
- Pound Play-Doh.
- Chop vegetables.
- Make pesto. (Cream that basil.)
- Get a job at a demolition site, or offer to volunteer with the sledge-hammer for an afternoon.
- Pull weeds.
- Scrub.
- Go for a run.
- Burn some incense.

I recently saw a play about the distinguished and twisted psychoanalyst Melanie Klein, and the coolest thing about this broad was that she had these three file drawers: The top one was for her super-ego— her bills and legal papers and such; the middle one was for her ego— manuscripts, letters, and all that; and then she had this wonderful bottom drawer that she kept locked—it was her "id drawer," and it held all the sordid, messed-up, shame-spiral material that we'd all rather keep locked up in our bodies.

Now, I feel pretty ill mentally at times, but you know whom I really worry about? After the moms I see at the bus stop threatening to bust their kids' head all over the cement? I worry about those moms for whom everything is always "great." Those moms who live in immaculate condos with white carpets, and, try as I might, I can't figure out where their id drawer is. See, there are those of us who are fucked up and know it, and those of us who are fucked up and don't know it. And I happen to think it's better to know it, and deal with it, long before that Pandora's box of wounding words gets so full it just bursts open and the shaming crap jumps from our lips and we find ourselves *becoming* that notorious woman at the bus stop we've all seen.

Parents' Rights

- You have the right not to be perfect.
- You have the right to put your own needs first sometimes.
- You have the right to express your feelings appropriately.
- You have the right to listen to Arrested Development at a reasonable volume.
- You have the right to ask for what you want or need.
- You have the right to your own opinions.
- You have the right to say no.
- You have the right not to be abused.
- You have the right to change your mind.
- You have the right to ask for help— emotional or practical.
- You have the right to eat spicy gumbo even if your kids think it smells nasty.
- You have the right to set limits and boundaries.
- You have the right to pursue your own interests and/or career.
- You have the right to take time for yourself.
- You have the right to have a social, romantic, and sexual life.
- You have the right to do a little jig whenever you want.

Children's Rights

- Children have the right to be children.
- Children have the right to be nurtured and cared for.
- Children have the right to express their feelings and ideas.
- Children have the right to listen to Raffi at a reasonable volume.
- Children have the right to ask for what they want or need.
- Children have the right to be believed.
- Children have the right to say no.
- Children have the right to be protected from abuse, neglect, and worries about grown-up problems.
- Children have the right not to have any idea who Rush Limbaugh is.
- Children have the right to be respected and accepted for who they are.
- Children have the right to have playmates and supportive grown-ups in their lives.
- Children have the right to know their limits and boundaries.
- Children have the right to make certain choices.
- Children have the right to natural consequences.
- Children have the right to privacy.
- Children have the right to do a little jig whenever they want.

Rebel Mom

Grandma Knows Best

Cherie McCoy, self-acceptance trainer, mother,
and grandmother of many

As a survivor of so many former toddlers, and with the work you do now, do you have any wisdom for those of us who are still in the trenches?

Children have to be allowed their "no." That is how they establish their autonomy. Often parents hear that "no" as a threat to their authority, or they don't allow the child their "no" because they smother them and say "You're a good girl" all of the time.

Between the ages of one and a half and three, two things are happening physically. The anal sphincter is developing and the corpus collasum in the brain is developing—so there are these changes at both ends of the body.

Children will potty train themselves unless they get into a power struggle over it. In my mother's day, you were really looked down upon if your child wasn't trained before he or she was a year old. It was like *you are not a good mother*. My mother is still so proud of the fact that by nine months I was walking to the potty and going. Little does she know what that does. There is a lot of self-loathing of the body that develops. Children who are forced to potty train— whether with praise or blame—tend to put on a lot of weight as adults, they grow up with a tight ass, and they tend to complain a lot. I love to complain. My mother used to say "You whine all the time," and of course I was complaining.

At the other end, in the brain, their autonomy is developing. For the first year and a half, the child is totally fused with the mother. The child feels what the mother feels. That's why when the mother is having a terrible day, the child will suddenly throw a tantrum, and the mother is thinking "Why today of all days?"

The other thing is that you have to be careful not to get into a power struggle. You have to be careful when you ask questions like "Do you want to go to bed now?" If you really want something from a child— this is where boundaries are—you don't ask a child. You just say "It's time for bed now."

I do believe in a five-minute warning and then you just pick them up and do a naptime ritual song as you put them in bed. Ritual is very important because it creates a sense of familiarity and safety.

I know you work with a lot of parents now, so I'm wondering how you help people deal with their anger and their rage.

A lot of us in our culture carry rage in our bodies—so what are we going to do with it? If we don't really work with ourselves, it's going to come out somewhere. Often we are mad at our own parents for what was done to us as children. I don't believe in going back to the actual parents and yelling at them—they were doing the best they could—but there are healthy ways to let that rage out, away from the child. When the child is absent, you can hit a pillow, or take a towel and wring it, or take a racket and hit something. You don't even need a racket if you can just feel it and breathe until it dissipates. There was a woman in one of my workshops the other day and she was all ready to hit with this racket, and I said, "Now, don't hit until you are really ready, and then hit and hit and don't stop." She was mad at her husband, so she was talking and yelling and then all of a sudden the rage went away. She just put down the racket and she didn't need to hit. It's just a tool so you can let that rage come up, and when you let it come up it's like an orgasm. It hits a peak and then it subsides and you feel cleansed.

The other thing about anger is that a lot of people become rage-a-holics. It becomes a habit—every time rage comes up, they yell and then they feel better. It actually lets loose endorphins, so they rage and rage, and then they feel good. That's fine if they've never raged before, but it's an awful habit to get into, it's like a drug.

What about when we blow it? I'm talking Bad Mother Days . . .

I think it's important, especially as children get older and they know that you blew it, to apologize. Even then, you don't do it right away. Wait until it's over and everything has calmed down. You don't want to get in the habit of raging and then apologizing all of the time.

The first time a child does something, I often see parents tell the child, "Stop doing that," and then they turn back and talk to their friend and then the child does it again and the parent says "I said stop doing that." They don't want to get up and go over and look in the child's eyes and say "What you are doing right now is not okay with me," and really give that child their full attention and look at her with calm but firm eyes rather than rageful eyes.

Now, it's important that mothers not use this information to judge themselves and beat themselves up. Our culture does not teach us how to be mothers, so all we have is what our mothers did to us. That's why I think it's so important to work on ourselves.

I've got this *Parenting Magazine* survey that says that half of American parents think they should hit their kids—at least spanking with their open hand— and that toddlers are the most likely victims. Do you think spanking or hitting is ever appropriate?

No, I don't. Children can be very trying, but I think it is abusive. [Spanking] is hitting right at the energy center, and it will create a blockage.

So what's the alternative?

The most effective discipline is taking your presence away from the child. That's why time-outs really do work if the parent does them in a calm way and doesn't leave the child too long. Really, one minute for every year the child is old. I've worked with people who were put in a room for days. That's horrible. What happens then is that the child is abandoned, which creates a whole other thing we could talk about. But you also can just say, "This is not okay, I am not allowing this." You can do that with your own children, and with other people's children.

Toddlerhood is a crazy, crazy time. But if we think about it, toddlerhood may have been the last time we were all our true selves—protesting every wrong, not wanting to share, rushing toward independence, but never forgetting that we needed someone to fall back on. "Little kids are assholes," Utah Philips says. "But they're their own assholes."

Chapter 5

Beauty and the Gender Beast

~~~~~~~~~~~~~~

*Adoring Barbie is a passing event rather than a
permanent condition.*

—*Sara Bonnet Stein,* The Limits of
Non-Sexist Child-rearing

"It's a baby!"

When's the last time you heard a gender-neutral birth
announcement? I think I've heard all of one in my life, and that was in
an essay, no doubt edited after the original words were uttered.

"Girls are impossible," my friend Marni tells me. "They know way
too much too fast."

"Boys are harder," another friend insists. "It's the testosterone."

"What if she's a girly girl?" my friend Nancy worries.

"What if he's totally out of control?" one dad wants to know.

Pink? Blue? Nonsexist yellow? Barbie? G.I. Joe? Androgynous rag
dolls? Whether we think there are any real differences between boys
and girls or not, gender matters. In a perfect world we could raise our
kids making adjustments only according to their temperaments and
our own. But there is another part of the equation. A part where gen-

der, race, and all of the differences our culture loves to emphasize are paramount.

"Up to about age two or three, they're unisex," Jennifer, a mother of two elementary school kids, tells me. "And then one day it hits them—I'm like my mom, or I'm not like my mom, and therefore I should be like Princess Diana or Sylvester Stallone."

Maia's first high-maintenance Princess Diana phase lasted only from about age three to five and then we seemed to be in the clear. But just the other day, my gorgeous soon-to-be seven-year-old looked in the mirror and said, "I don't like my face. I look like a boy."

I took a deep breath and jumped back into the ring. Fighting sexism and all the blows to my daughter's self-esteem, I sometimes feel like I'm up against Mike Tyson himself, and I'm down for the count more often than not. But we all learn to fight and defend against the gender beast one round at a time, and unlike professional boxers, we're allowed to hit below the belt and do whatever it takes to kick the dominant culture's ass.

Just to get you started, here are a few Hip Mama strategies for nonsexist child rearing.

Point Out the Bearded Lady

Lee Johnson, an acquaintance of mine who passed away a few years ago, was my nonsexist child-rearing idol. I didn't have the chance to get to know her very well, but the few conversations I had with Lee rocked my world. She was a family therapist and lesbian mom with a little boy, and she had learned to be daring in teaching her child what was what. Just as some parents help their kids to think of opposites as they are learning about the language and the concept, Lee played "the Stereotype Game" with her son. After explaining the idea to him, they played like this:

"It's a stereotype that girls can't play football as well as boys. Try to think of a stereotype."

"Kids can't fly."

"Good. But usually kids *can't* fly. Can you think of any stereotypes that aren't true?"

"Boys are poop-heads. Is that a stereotype?"

"Yes. That's a stereotype."

"And boys are mean. That's a stereotype. But sometimes boys *are* mean."

"Yep. But it's a stereotype to say that *all* boys are mean."

"All girls are nice, that's a stereotype."

"Yes."

"And yellow hair is nicer, that's a stereotype. And monsters are scary. Is that a stereotype?"

You've gotta love it. In a commentary Lee once wrote for *Hip Mama*, she talked about snatching up every little opportunity our kids give us for these kinds of lessons. "The only way kids can learn new things is through their immediate experiences," she wrote. So when an immediate experience presented itself, she jumped at the opportunity to teach the lesson.

As Lee was standing in line at the grocery store with her son one day, she noticed a guy wearing a lesbian T-shirt. Intrigued, she took another look. It was actually a woman with a full beard. "How'd you do that?" Lee asked.

"Easy," the woman said. "I just stopped shaving."

Lee knew very well that some women tweezed and shaved their facial hairs, but it had never occurred to her that a woman could grow a full beard. She made sure her son noticed the bearded woman too.

"The idea that women can never have beards must be a stereotype," her six-year-old son told her, unfazed.

Another time, Lee's eight-year-old neighbor admitted to being upset that she couldn't figure out if another person on the block was a man or a woman.

"That's okay," Lee reassured her. "They're androgynous-looking." And the girl was quite satisfied with this new concept.

When my daughter, then four, saw a picture on the front page of the newspaper of two men getting married, she laughed. She had been to several same-sex weddings when she was younger, but now she told me, "Two men can't get married."

It was time for a lesson.

"Concepts are never too hard to grasp if they are tied in with immediate sensory experiences," according to Lee. "The concepts we learn empower us, even when there are a lot of syllables involved."

Free Polly Pocket

Every time I wind up in K-Mart or some similar toy hell, I'm amazed that they still divide up all the toys not by age-appropriateness but by gender. There's the pink aisle with Barbie and Ken getting married in a box. (They don't tell kids the part where Ken comes out, introduces his boyfriend to the family, and the lovely couple has to get a divorce.) And then there's the primary-colors aisle with all the balls and weapons. I mean, what year is it? Aren't we over this? Well, the dominant culture certainly isn't. And as usual, it's us moms who have to deal with the fallout.

When I was little, my mother's reaction to all of this was simply not to buy any crap. "Commercialism is like a vacuum," she would tell me. "It will suck you up." She had a long list of these somewhat dramatic warnings—"Don't be the kind of girl who screams in biology class," and "Don't lose track of what's beautiful and what's plastic." It was 1975. I was five years old. And feminism had met the toy industry.

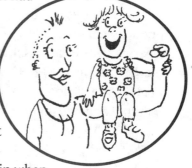

I don't remember owning even a single plastic doll (but I do remember all the cool stuff my friends had). Yes, I may have grown up to be a feminist, but as a guinea pig in the great experiment of nonsexist child rearing of the 1970s, I felt utterly deprived.

I started tripping on the toy industry again when Maia was a toddler. I knew I didn't have it in me to ban Barbie and all the other junk in the pink aisle, but I wanted to find some kind of balance—some kind of maternal feminism that wouldn't make her feel too deprived.

"Censoring can create something forbidden and they begin to think it must be really exciting," agreed Holly Gordon, a psychotherapist and feminist psychology professor I consulted on my quest for nonsexist balance. "But what you *can* do is promote critical thinking in terms of gender."

When Maia stood before me in a pink dress and, pushing her bangs out of her face, said, "I wish I could be the real Snow White," Holly suggested I ask, "Do you think it would be fun staying home and cooking for all those dwarfs?"

"It doesn't mean that you can't have an opinion about [the toys] once you've elicited theirs," she told me. "Sometimes it's more important for children to feel that you respect their choices and how they want to present themselves."

I buy some of the crap Maia sees on TV, but I've learned to point it out when the toys turn out to be bogus. And instead of dissing K-Mart altogether, I've learned to shop in both aisles. She doesn't have any guns (I do draw the line there, all right?), but she's got balls, swords, train sets, and buckets of Star Wars action figures as well as the dolls and baking sets she insists she *must have*.

Don't get me wrong now. I don't hold *all* of my feminist commentary in favor of therapeutically correct questions without judgments. Whenever I see one of those weird muffins that turns into a sexy little doll, I tell all the children in the vicinity to repeat after mama: "Women are not baked goods."

The other day when Maia and her friends were lamenting the predicament of a "Polly Pocket" doll that had been sealed inside a clear plastic dome by some deranged toy designer, I wielded the hammer that ultimately freed her. (If you haven't had the pleasure, "Polly Pocket" is a strange little plastic woman who is about a quarter of an inch tall and has no nose, which is better than "Hello Kitty," who has no mouth.)

And whenever I hear a conversation turn to *Beauty and the Beast*, I remind everyone within earshot that the story is make-believe—in real life, beasts will be beasts no matter how long you stay with them.

We can't pretend that the world will be any kinder to our daughters than it has been to us—in some ways it will be, and in some ways it will not be—but we can do our best to help our girls hang on to that natural, "Harriet the Spy," kick-butt spirit they are born with. There will be days when they look in the mirror and say "I don't like my face," but if we deal with it head on, right when we hear it, then I honestly believe we can do a lot to arm them against all the garbage the world has waiting for them.

In *Reviving Ophelia*, Mary Pipher notes that while many of us worry about sex stereotyping when our daughters are small, we often throw in the (Little Mermaid) towel all too soon. The time to really worry is early adolescence, Pipher tells us, but perhaps we can support our daughters in "resisting the cultural definitions of femininity" right through their childhoods—playing it by ear, giving a little here, winging it a little there, but remaining basically steadfast in our support and our belief in them as people.

As one mama says, "We act like that self-esteem crisis just appears out of nowhere when our kids are teenagers, but really it's something that's been happening all along. The symptoms might not show up until our girls are older, but I think if we are really checking in with them, really helping them heal whatever blows to their confidence are going on, then we can head off a lot of the problems."

If all else fails (well, even if it doesn't), it might just cheer you up to remember the Barbies and Kens "to Come" featured in an early issue of the New York City zine *Hey There Barbie Girl!* Mattel eventually stopped the zine from being published, but, just for old times' sake: There was *Totally Cockring Ken* "check out that jacket!"; *Psycho Ex-boyfriend Ken* "Restraining orders not included, but strongly suggested"; *Bi-lingual Administrative Assistant Barbie* who could say "Get your own damn coffee" in three languages; and the ever-popular *Non-stop Talking Barbie* who "doesn't shut up until you break her damn head off." Add those to the *Trailer Park Barbie* and *Androgynous Kerbie* dolls already on our Christmas wish lists, and we might just be able to work with the mainstream culture.

Mission Impossible?

Game Plan	Probable Result
Sew black power symbol on all garments, only read bedtime stories from *Ms.* and *Socialist Worker*, decorate nursery with posters of *Rosey the Riveter*, *Che Guevara*, *Mao Zedong*, and *Lorena Bobbit*.	Difficult teen years blamed on "weird hippie parents," joins ROTC but grows up to lead military coup against the U.S. government.

Paint nursery pink for a girl named "Muffy," buy only Barbie-related toys, shame child when she asks for any variety or expresses any independent feelings.	Miss America who gains worldwide fame but is stripped of her title when *Playboy* spread comes out.
Paint nursery blue for a boy named "Grunt," buy only guns and trucks, shame child when he asks for any variety or expresses any nurturing feelings.	Militia leader who gains worldwide fame but is stripped of his position when *Playgirl* spread comes out.
Name child "Pat," paint nursery yellow, and when s/he asks anything related to gender, say "I told you, gender is a social construction, goddammit!"	Difficult teen years blamed on "weird hippie parents"; after $5,000 in gender confusion therapy lands starring role making fun of you on *Saturday Night Live*.
Wing it: Name kid Tony or Toni, paint room yellow, offer a variety of toys, sew black power symbol on some garments, deal with issues as they arise, offer frequent feminist commentary.	Short-lived backlash during teen years blamed on "weird feminist parents"; after $5,000 in therapy dealing with other issues, grows up to found Feminist Party, landing first radical babe in White House.

Negotiate a Testosterone Truce

"This might sound sexist," one mama tells me, "but I have to have more boundaries with my son and more cheering on with my daughter because I know that teachers and society in general are going to place more limits on my girl. I'm not talking about oppressing my son so it will be even, I'm talking about focusing on the parts of my kids that the greater world will ignore—and those parts are different for boys and girls. Let's be real: If my daughter comes home with a shiner, it'll probably be because she wasn't quite big enough for the situation; if my son comes home with a shiner, it might just be because he was a little too big."

Another friend agrees, but only partly. "You have to be careful with that kind of thinking," she says. "If we agree that misogyny begins with a kind of jealousy of girl-culture, then, as a parent, I want to be extra careful that my boys don't feel that they are missing out on something. That will just make them resentful."

It's a dilemma most mothers of sons find themselves in sooner or later—when infant androgyny blossoms into toddler testosterone.

"I'm gonna be mean when I get big," Tim says. "I'm gonna be The Man."

"Lovely" is the only reaction his mother can conjure at first, but every woman alive knows the images that started to race through this mama's head. The blueprint for self-destruction and male privilege society hands our sons is at least as scary as the legacy dumped on our daughters. It's different, but it's just as scary. And as women, we often feel ill-equipped to help our boys reject that blueprint.

One mom I know got into a spot when she decided that her home needed to be a little more "male-friendly." It started when her son objected to some feminist folk music she was playing, and she panicked—would he grow up to hate women? Would he grow up feeling like his maleness "wasn't being honored"?

She started looking around for more positive images of men she thought would make life better for her son, but there simply weren't many to choose from. I suggested posters of Martin Luther King, Jr., Caesar Chavez, Che Guevara, even Bill Nye the Science Guy from PBS. "Yeah," she agreed. "But I was thinking of art. I was thinking of something like the equivalent of Frida Kahlo, and there just isn't that much."

True, but we have to take what we can get: posters, whatever art with images of "positive maleness" we can find, and, perhaps, a more relaxed approach to the whole question. As my friend well knows, men are not born batterers, they have to go through some pretty serious hell to become that hateful and messed up. I don't want to dump the responsibility of raising "good sons" all on moms (rather than on the culture that actually encourages our kids to become angry and hateful), but there is plenty of damage control we can do with our boys.

In the beginning we may be dealing with relatively simple stuff. Most of us, for example, don't have any problem dressing our girls in blue—or whatever—and only my grandma flinched when Maia's favorite toy was a train set. But what about the boys? It still makes a lot of folks nervous to see a little guy in a pink sleeper. "William Wants a Doll" was all good and fine in the '70s, but a lot of us still flinch when Johnny wants to be the princess. So we have to begin by stripping our minds of all of these prejudices.

Lindsay, the mother of a five-year-old boy, says her biases come out as she tries to deal with her children's emotions. "I've noticed that mothers of girls sometimes don't have as much trouble letting their kids express their emotions, whether they are sadness, anger, joy, or whatever. With Jake, I'm always tempted to say 'Oh, be brave,' or I'm tempted to be more afraid of his anger and say 'Get a hold of yourself,' it takes a lot of patience for me to remember that he needs to let those emotions fly, as long as he's not hurting anyone."

I know one first grader who, although he has never appeared to have any shortage of testosterone pulsing through his veins, has his drag queen days. His mom is a very cool chick who doesn't say a word until he wants to go out, at which point she kindly warns him that even though he looks fabulous, "Some people might make fun of you. Some people are *like that*." So this kid knows what's up. I've seen him running down the sidewalk after an ice cream truck all decked out in a princess outfit and my daughter's choker necklace, but he wears khakis and T-shirts to school. School always has a disproportionate number of people who are "like that," he explains. And he'll only set himself up for as much ridicule as he can deal with.

As the poet Audre Lorde put it, "The strongest lesson I can teach my son is the same lesson I can teach my daughter: how to be who he wishes to be for himself. And the best way I can do this is to be who I am and hope he will learn from this not how to be me, which is impossible, but how to be himself. And this means how to move to that voice from within himself, rather than to those raucous, persuasive, or threatening voices from the outside, pressuring him to be what the world wants him to be."

Decolonize Your Brain

I once edited a commentary that Joy Viveros wrote about her son and children of color in general. "Do I see aggressive behavior in a child of color as showing evidence of potential to be a great lawyer or a great street thug?" she suggested we all ask ourselves. And her little test stuck with me. When I know I'm dealing with the gender beast—or the race beast, or any other beast—I pause and ask myself: *Would I feel differently if she were a boy? Would I say something else if he were white? What if he was a Latino? Would I tell him "no" then?* We all need to be sure we are being culturally sensitive, but just as the biggest difference between boys and girls is how we treat them, the biggest difference between people of different races, sexual preferences, cultural backgrounds, and classes is how we react to them. As Maya Angelou puts it, "We are more alike, my friends, then we are unalike."

Obviously, racism and sexism are different beasts. Sometimes we meet them together—as one mother of an African-American boy says, "We all have been socialized to see my cute little son as a monster." Sometimes we meet them separately. But, as we are raising our children, many of the same issues, problems, and solutions can be applied whether we are talking about misogyny, race-hatred, classism, homophobia, or any other kind of bigotry.

Just as mothers of sons have to figure out how to unpack the male privilege diaper bag, the parents among us raising European American kids can't ignore the racism beast. It haunts us all, and we will all be called upon to, as they say "comfort the afflicted and afflict the comfortable."

Coming Soon to a Theater Near You

Snow White and the Seven Patriarchs

The Bigot King

Codependent and the Beast

Unconscious Beauty

The Little Mermute

One important strategy to remember when we are dealing with any of the "isms" is that we should comfort the victim of the insults or injuries before we deal with the source. If your child gets knocked off his bike, you make sure he is all right before you go after the bully, right? And so when we see the racism beast bite, we should first do our best to tend to the wounds of the child of color. Then we can educate the source of his injury by pointing out stereotypical comments, teaching him the history of bigotry and the civil rights movement, and staging mass actions against the powers that encourage intolerance.

All of this begins with working on ourselves and our own stereotypes. We have to strip our minds of our unfair imaginings about "the others" as well as internalized stereotypes about ourselves and those "like us." But do not be afraid to fight the "isms" in the world even before you feel you have completely decolonized your own mind. These are processes that can occur simultaneously—teaching our children, teaching our culture, and teaching ourselves.

Tell the Ad Wizards Where to Go

Here's an average baby product ad: a picture of an androgynous-looking infant and the text, "Soon enough there'll be ballet lessons and boys at the front door. But for now, Johnson's Baby her." As we start to get acquainted with the gender beast, these things seem more and more obnoxious. Who's to say she won't be taking kickboxing lessons or there won't be baby dykes at the door?

Please make a thousand copies of the note to the left and just keep the stack on your desk. Whenever you see a ridiculous ad, rip it out and send it back with your note to the ad wizards who saw fit to create it.

> ### This Promotes Stereotypes
>
> *Please let me know when you decide to end this line of*
>
> ❏ *sexist* ❏ *racist*
> ❏ *classist* ❏ *homophobic*
>
> *advertising and I will resume buying your product.*

If you have the time and the inclination, more in-depth feedback is always good too. I know a mama who actually got a big diaper company to stop printing little white heterosexual nuclear families on their training pants with a well-thought-out letter. Oftentimes these ad wizards just aren't thinking, and if they hear rumblings about a boycott, they may very well change their tune.

Nostalgic? '70s Babes Remember Our Own Youth

"I got my period when I was eleven and my mom wanted to throw a party to celebrate my womanhood. I was horrified. I just wanted to go to the Emporium and buy some new pants and she wanted to celebrate my womanhood."
—Selene, thirty

"I don't believe there was a single doll in my room. I got this perfume for Christmas once and I smashed it in the street. But you know what? I put a little perfume on before I smashed it. I was secretly into it."   —Melissa, twenty-nine

"My mom was cool. She was like, this is how you treat women. When I was in high school, my girlfriend called me a male-chauvinist pig and my mom said she was right. I was a little upset about that, I mean, I kind of thought my mom should be on my side. But maybe they were right."
—Marco, twenty-seven

"What can I say? Mixed feelings. There were days when I just wanted my mom in the kitchen baking cookies like a normal mom, but looking back, the fact that she worked and organized and lived the way she wanted to live made me who I am. I wouldn't have had it any other way."
—Sarah, twenty-five

Do as You Say

All right, now. Have you got a man and a woman in your household? Who does the dishes? Who works outside the home? Who takes out the garbage? Who changes the oil in the car? Who takes care of baby when he's feeling under the weather? It's all right if you already know you're failing this little quiz, but we have to watch out if we're teaching nonsexism without modeling it.

How's dad at nurturing? How's mom at sticking up for what she needs and wants? Say mom stays home and dad works—nothing wrong with that, as long as everyone's pleased with the setup, and mom still gives herself the room to pursue her dreams. Any lifestyle and any equal division of labor a couple decides on can work, but when the gender beast rears its ugly head in our own lives—especially when we're deciding how to set up shop for a kid—it's important for us to give ourselves the same guidance we would like to offer our youngsters.

In generations past, a lot of women felt as if they had to stay in patriarchal marriages "for the sake of the children." Feminism has taught us, however, that it doesn't do our kids any good to watch us being oppressed. Even when the issues we face are seemingly "less serious," we do need to treat ourselves the way we would like to see our sons and daughters treated.

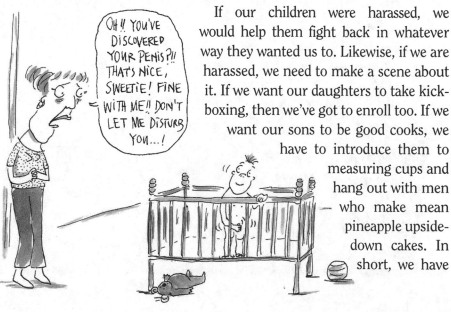

If our children were harassed, we would help them fight back in whatever way they wanted us to. Likewise, if we are harassed, we need to make a scene about it. If we want our daughters to take kickboxing, then we've got to enroll too. If we want our sons to be good cooks, we have to introduce them to measuring cups and hang out with men who make mean pineapple upside-down cakes. In short, we have to *become* the role models we wish we could find for our children.

I myself didn't become a radical feminist until after my daughter was born. Sure, I had always been a bleeding heart liberal—when I was fifteen I was out there in front of the federal building in San Francisco raising the Sandinista flag and blockading the entrance in some kind of bizarre attempt to tell the U.S. government to get out of Central America. I had been a feminist too, but my *radical* feminist agenda came later. There were times during my postbaby transformation when I felt like becoming empowered "for the sake of my daughter" was just about as stereotypically femme as I could get. We are, after all, supposed to become empowered for *ourselves*, aren't we? But I've since decided that it doesn't really matter what it takes for us to start grabbing the patriarchy by its throat and screaming epithets. Some of the women in my kickboxing class, I am sure, started training because they thought the exercise would make them fit for a Calvin Klein ad. Well, so what? No matter what their motivation, they will learn to kick some ass.

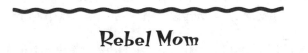

Rebel Mom

The Deal with Testosterone

Mary Kay Blakely, feminist writer mom, author of
American Mom *and* Red, White and Oh So Blue

So, what's the deal with testosterone?

It is a major force in the universe, isn't it? When my sons were both really little, I thought that there was not much difference at that stage between male and female. I mean, the cultural influences are overwhelming right from the beginning, and kids pick up the cues from everywhere, but when a child hasn't learned speech, the whole repertoire of emotions are there in both genders.

It begins to emerge big time in preadolescence. By that time social conditioning has taken over. My son Darren, particularly, felt that because he didn't play sports, what was there to be proud of? He did learn to play sports in high school, and it was important to him to do that, to find the part of himself that hauls ass and bangs away out on the field. But it was astonishing to me, growing up in the household he grew up in, that he would be able to say something like "What's good about me? I don't even play sports."

But you didn't notice that until they started getting older?

I do have to say, even when they were really tiny kids, we said, "Okay, no war toys in the house, no guns," but what would be the first thing they would build with their Lego blocks or Tinker Toys? Guns. I couldn't tell you whether that was a male thing. I guess it is. I don't know that girls build many guns. But what are all the images from cartoons? From TV? Even if you don't have guns in your house, you're going to walk by twenty thousand posters of Arnold Schwarzenegger in the mall, so they do pick up, *This is male, this is brave, this is honorable.*

I don't think that anything we do as parents in that regard begins to counter the cultural influences, it just gives them another whole plethora of ideas to use along with what they learn from the culture.

I was talking to another single mother of sons the other day. She's very female-centered and a very strong feminist, but she is worried that maybe her sons are going to grow up feeling as if their home wasn't a place where their maleness was welcomed and honored, you know?

My kids both felt that. It took me a while to understand that it was important for me to be in the bleachers watching the football games. I did not understand how important that part of their world was to them. Like with Ryan, it was through wrestling that he found the key to his own self-discipline and drive, and it just gave him enormous confidence. He found a really safe arena in which to explore the part of himself that wanted to pound another guy into the floor. He definitely experienced pain, I couldn't stand it when I watched, but for him it was a necessary thing to do. It was a somewhat alienating experience for me to be in the bleachers because I did not introduce him to this very important part of himself; he discovered it on his own, and my role was to figure out *How do I recognize what it is for him and celebrate it when it is so outside my world?* But then you do enter the other culture and figure out what's good and what's bad. I also felt like it was okay that I wasn't the major cheerleader for that part of him, because there were coaches and so many other people.

A lot of moms I know have this sense that they know what they want for their girls, but they're a little less confident with the boys. . . .

There is a serious shortage of male feminist heroes. We can promote aggressive behavior in our daughters and we can promote ambition in our daughters because we feel it will be used in healthy and useful directions. We are more reluctant to encourage that in our male children, because all the venues they have for that are venues that have oppressed us.

It's hard for us to point to men now who are actively changing the culture. They do all kinds of work in the antiwar movement and in the civil rights movement, but they don't make the link to the women's movement.

I think that's something that mothers are going to keep wrestling with until society changes. Children may have their dads, and they may have friends of the family, but in terms of cultural images, what do we have? We have *Mr. Mom*, which is a comedy. You only see feminist men in the culture as wimps or comics. I don't mind comedy at all, but there are many more images of strong women that we can enthusiastically give to our daughters.

Do you have any more advice for mothers of very young kids?

At that stage, I say full throttle ahead with feminism! When they are that young, you still have lots of influence over them. It gets subtracted a little bit more every year, so everything that you plant in there in those early ages is exceedingly valuable, and you don't have to worry about "overdoing it" because you are up against the entire culture.

As we move forward full throttle with maternal feminism, can I offer a little product endorsement? Remember that Marlo Thomas album *Free to be You and Me?* I recently picked it up in vinyl, but they've got it on CD too. And if you ask me, it's still the best kid's collection ever produced. Remember Carol Channing doing her little spoken word piece about how no one likes housework? Or Rosey Grier singing "It's All Right to Cry"? Stop me before I melt into total 1972 tofu-baby nostalgia, but if you were raised by a bunch of hippies like I was, you too will find yourself dancing around the house with your kids and singing along . . .

Chapter 6

Finding Your Village

~~~~~~~~~~~~~~~~~~~~~~~~~~~~~

If it takes a village to raise a child, where is my village? —*Opal Palmer Adisa, novelist*

When my friend Shana remarried, she and her husband decided it was time to buy a new home. After looking at housing prices in the city where they both lived and where Shana ran a single-mother support group, they decided they would have to move to a new town. After a lot of searching, they bought a house they both loved in a sub- urban area they thought would be nice for their son. But as the family settled in and started meeting their new neighbors, Shana was sure they'd moved to hell.

"The other moms were like 'What? You nurse? That's so gross.' And they kept telling me I should spank the baby when he cried," she said. "I'd built this whole community before we moved, and suddenly I had no one."

Shana called her old friends a lot, but phone calls weren't enough. Finally a friend suggested that she call La Leche League. At least the mothers there would believe in nursing, her friend reminded her.

The closest La Leche League group was a half-hour drive from where Shana lived, but she started making the drive and began to create a new community of mothers she could talk to, hang out with, and call for baby-sitting and other help. Some of the women in the group, to Shana's surprise, even lived in her new neighborhood.

While some women go through their pregnancies and early years of motherhood surrounded by like-minded friends, most of us have to go out of our way to find that vital village of support.

A friend with a six-month-old baby recently walked into a solstice party at my house looking pale and confused. I offered her a drink and as she sat down on the couch, she looked up at me and said, slowly, "Wait. Culture shock. Let me adjust." She could not remember the last time she was at a party. She adjusted though, and by the end of the night she admitted, "I didn't realize how much I missed people—how much I missed myself."

Don't Even Think about Staying Home with the Curtains Drawn

It's probably going to happen at some point. You get a divorce and discover that 90 percent of your "friends" are on such shaky ground in their own marriages that they can't even talk to you. You have a new baby and start to notice that all of your old buddies spend their nonworking hours at the bar. You move to a new place and every mom in your trailer park looks like June Cleaver on a bad hair day. Or you wake up one morning to find that you have drifted away from every supportive friend you ever had.

When you find yourself feeling alone, take heart—there are kindred spirits out there. Don't even think about staying home with the curtains drawn, or you will soon find yourself going completely insane, calling the three-dollar-a-minute psychic hot line for hours on end—or worse, inviting those nice Jehovah's Witnesses in for tea.

So get out, already. Go to the park, go to your local café, find a La Leche League meeting in your area, go to your local senior center and adopt a grandparent if you don't have enough cool family members around, sign up for a class, check the "Bulletin Board" section in your community newspaper for support groups, call one of the national support group referral centers listed in the back of this book, advertise about starting a new group, subscribe to on-line and print zines that are still small enough to feel like a family: *Welfare Mother's Voice, Biracial Child, SingleMOTHER, Hip Mama, Sage Woman, HUES, Bust* . . . whatever!

I could tell you about a million other places to go, publications to read, and things to do to start finding your village, but I don't think it would be terribly helpful. There are really only two things you have to remember when you feel like you are becoming isolated.

The first is that you do have to get out—you have to reach out, you have to make human contact. I know one woman who lives way out in the middle of nowhere in Canada's Yukon. The winters are long and dark and the closest town is very small. She and her young daughter are totally isolated. But they are not alone. In town, they have met a few friends, and they cherish those connections. She subscribes to zines also, but human contact—the friend who invites them over for dinner or the mile-away neighbor who stops by with some firewood— is all-important. No matter where you live, you have to get out and make the sometimes Herculean effort.

The second thing is that you have to be yourself. It sounds simple, and obvious, but sometimes this is where we get stuck. As much as we want to "fit in" with whatever group seems the most convenient to connect with (Hey, the Jehovah's Witnesses make *house calls*), we soon find out that a bunch of cheesy, bogus friends whom we have to put on airs for just to hang out with does not a village make. Sure, sometimes the ladies at Gymboree are better than no one, and we often find that we have a lot more in common with those big-haired June Cleaver chicks than we thought we did. But let's face it, if you can't fart around your friends, you're just not a whole lot better off than you were staying home with your curtains drawn.

This village I'm talking about doesn't have to be huge. One good friend—preferably one with kids—whom you can pick your nose in front of will do. Having two or three of these babes whom you can hang out with on a somewhat regular basis is fabulous. Throw in a once-a-month support group where you can cry, and this thing is starting to look like a real village.

I say it's preferable that at least some of these folks have children not only because they give your kid someone to play with, but because sometimes only another mama really *gets* the meaning of sleep depri-vation. But we don't have to diss everyone without children. Even when our kids are really young, our *whole* lives don't have to revolve around them. And a lot of people without kids do like having them around. Julia is one of my dependable village babes—she doesn't have kids of her own yet, but she's totally into my daughter. When Maia got sick on a day when I just knew I wasn't going to be able to handle it alone, I just bundled her up and headed over to Julia's house. We talked, Maia slept, and Julia—not worn out by kids of her own and not terribly worried about anyone in her household catching the flu—made us soup.

It can take some time to find a group of people—a chosen family—you can count on. Like "The Ugly Duckling" or my friend in the Yukon, you may find that it is a long, long winter, but no matter where you live in the world, there really are folks out there.

Jessica, one of my childhood friends, used to say something like "I have a million friends, I just haven't met them all yet." And she was right. I swear I won't make fun of you if you repeat this line like a daily affirmation whenever you're feeling alone in the world.

Old Friends, New Friends

One of the most surprising things about becoming a mom, says Ali, a thirty-year-old married gal, was "finding out which friends stuck by me and which friends either felt jealous of the time I spent with my son or couldn't relate to me anymore." Our circles of friends are always changing, but there's nothing like having a baby to totally shake up your social scene. The first few years of parenthood make our lives so child-centered that many of our old connections just seem to fizzle out. But new connections do arise.

Support Groups

I just ran out to my local café and picked up all the community newspapers. Here are a few of the things I found: a monthly social group for gay and lesbian parents of color, an Asian-American women's group, an information and support group for new moms, a therapy group for women going through divorce, a play group for toddlers, a support group for children going through divorce, and a mom's hiking group. I also found a lot of ads for penis enlargement and dolphin chanting, but whatever.

Even if there aren't as many groups in your area, that's no excuse—you can start one. I read recently that about one third of all Americans belong to some kind of support or therapy group. So, really now, it's not just the New Agers. There are all kinds of "recovery" groups out there, which can be great, but I'm talking here about mutual support and social groups—places where you can make friends, process experiences, talk about your kids, and share your stresses. You may want to begin by just advertising about *wanting* to start a group and see if you can't find a couple of radical babes to help you out. If you don't want to do the formal thing, you may want to start getting together with all your interested acquaintances on a regular basis. One mama I know has a sort of open-house coffee thang every Saturday morning. It's somewhat high maintenance to swear you'll always be home and have coffee, but it can be fun. Besides, this woman just has a shortage of time, not really a shortage of friends. Having them all over at once is one way she can deal with staying connected.

> ## Some Signs That You Need to Get Out More . . .
>
> - You are beginning to think of someone you only know as "yip34@zap.com" as one of your closest friends.
> - You send yourself mail just so you can chat with the mail delivery babe.
> - You have been wearing the same electric blue fuzzy robe your mother gave you for Christmas for seven days straight and there is nothing physically wrong with you.
> - You honestly couldn't summarize the local weather pattern over the past few days.
> - You talk to the guy who calls with the Toyota marketing survey—for an hour.
> - You have found yourself lately pondering your spiritual connection with Montel Williams.

If you are going to start a formal support group and you've found a couple of other people to help you, you'll probably want to start by deciding what the focus and purpose of the group is going to be. Are you looking for feminist moms, new moms, mothers and daughters, queer moms, single parents, black women, feminists with or without kids, green-haired bisexual mothers of one-year-olds? Your group can be as specific or as general as you want it to be, but you do have to think about the purpose of your group. Do you want to relax and have potlucks with like-minded parents? Do you want to talk about specific issues? Do you want a play group for your kids? Do you want revolutionary coconspirators? Do you want it all?

A good way to begin is to go to a few existing groups in your area, even if they are not exactly the gang you are looking for. You can see how they operate and talk to people about starting groups, about what works, and about what doesn't. Yes, ladies, I'm talking about *networking*. Even if you don't end up starting a group, I've already got you off your butt, down to the café, and maybe even off to a meeting.

There are, of course, little oddities you have to deal with on the support-group circuit, but mostly, parents report getting a lot out of their regular meetings. As my single dad friend says, "It's really nice just to go and have someone else look after Tony and relax with a bunch of other people who don't ask where his mom is and aren't always hassling me about *how I do it*." Sure, there are always going to be the folks in the circle who are totally whiny and needy and weird, but you get to a point where you don't let them dominate everything, and you discover that even *their* realities are supportable.

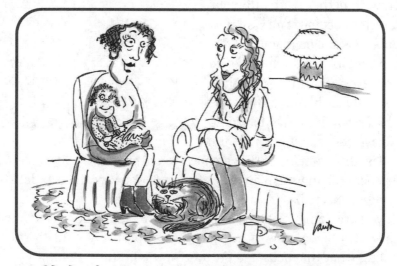

"She has finally surpassed the cat in intelligence."

Get Over It: Five Girls You Will Meet (or, Perhaps, Be) on the Mother's Support Group Circuit

Cat Mama: "I don't have any children, but I'm here because I really feel I have the same kinds of issues with my cat, whose name is Faye Dunaway."

Whiner Mama: "I'm here because, well, I'm just feeling *reeaally* stressed out and alone in dealing with my *Los Angeles Times* subscription renewal."

Psycho Ball of Issues Mama: "Every time I look into my infant son's eyes, I just see this big green hairy frightening monster, and then I think back to my own father, and then I remember the day last year when I tried to kill my neighbor's cat and I painted my bedroom with Liquid Paper, and then I just think I should move in with my therapist. . . . By the way, is anyone interested in cohousing?"

Super-Organized Mama: "All right, now that we've all introduced ourselves, let's break up into small groups. Group number one will be in charge of planning co-op grocery shopping, group number two should plan our weekly excursions for the next six months, group number three will create a new-member questionnaire . . ."

Cooler-Than-You Mama: "I just came by to check out the scene. It's been real. . . ."

Co-op Parenting

When I moved into family housing on the Mills College campus, I discovered a very cool extension of the traditional support group—a posse of moms who traded baby-sitting, meals, transportation, and the occasional boyfriend. I've since met a lot of families who do the co-op parenting thing. Some live miles apart but share certain child-rearing responsibilities. Others bring the idea of the Israeli kibbutz or the '60s commune home and live in rural communities, urban housing clusters, or in one big old hippie house. When I left Mills, I moved into a apartment upstairs from Julie, one of the moms from the Mills posse who had graduated the year before. We continued the co-op, sharing meals, baby-sitting, and transportation, and over the months and years, several other families have joined us and moved on.

Ken Norwood, an architect and founder of the Shared Living Resource Center in Berkeley, California, is one of the visionaries at the forefront of the post-1960s cooperative living movement. He is especially down with the idea of the "Village Cluster"—folks getting together and moving into the same building, block, or neighborhood to create intentional communities. "From studying indigenous people and their villages, both historic and present, it is clear to me that the tribe, clan, extended family, village, family farm, church, and town/neighborhood served instinctual survival needs for the growth and sustainability of cultures." Norwood writes in his book, *Rebuilding Community in America*. "I envision society re-adopting the historic patterns of human settlement and creating modern-day villages, extended family households, and family compounds."

You can give the Shared Living Resource Center a call at (510) 548-6608 to find out more about community and co-op living. They have enough information and resources to bury an army.

I may be something of a commitment-phobe, but I want to warn you to be really careful about jumping into any co-op living or parenting arrangement that would be difficult to pull out of. Like any partnership, you have to know that the families you get together with are on the same page as you are in terms of parenting, discipline philosophies, and general worldview. Make a list of the things that are important to you in child care, food, housing, and anything else you are planning to do cooperatively. The adults in your child's life don't all have to be like you, you just need to share the basics. Julie, my friend who lives in my building and with whom I've co-op parented since we met at Mills, has some different rules in her house than I have in mine. We have different TV policies, different temperaments, and different opinions about how often we should order pizza on our dinner nights. But these things are minor. Our kids know what's up, and they play us for it sometimes, but we agree on the important things.

No matter what you are doing cooperatively, agree to check in with your other group members on a regular basis. If you start feeling like you've got the short end of a deal, speak up. There's nothing like built-up resentment to destroy a perfectly cool co-op. Keep track of what everyone is doing. This does not have to be terribly strict and military—some parents use poker chips or Popsicle sticks as currency and agree on the relative values of what they put into the cooperative to make sure no one is getting stuck with all the baby-sitting while everyone else is off at Lollapalooza.

Julie and I have talked about taking our co-op one step further and getting a big house to share, but we both know that cohousing is a much more complicated thing to pull off than living in the same building but being able to retreat, when necessary, to our own spaces. When families share a home, every adult really does become something of a parent to all the children. You have to think about all the roommate questions you've always had to ponder. (Who does the dishes? What to do about weird boyfriends and relatives? Does anyone mind listening to Jill Sobule music?) And then you've got the parenting stuff to deal with. (How long do time-outs last? How do we all feel about Jim Carrey movies? Do we ever resort to hitting? If one adult says "no," is that the end of it? Are some kids allowed to eat chocolate and others not?) It gets complicated, but the rewards are often well worth the trouble.

As Tomasa, a mom who lives cooperatively with two other families, says, "Of course we have problems. Any big, extended family does. But this one of my choosing beats the hell out of my biological family."

Rebel Mom

Commie Mommy

Jessica Mitford (a.k.a. Decca Treuhaft), former
Communist Party member; muckracker extraordinaire;
lead singer, Decca and the Dectones; author of
The American Way of Death, The American Way of Birth,
and other books. (Six months after this interview, Jessica
Mitford died of lung cancer at the age of seventy-nine.)

You've always been very politically active, how was that when your children were young—being an activist mama?

When there was a Communist Party, the feeling was that everything you did in the direction of progress would somehow lead toward a revolution. I was, for example, the cookie chairman of the PTA. Honestly, I was. Our son Benjamin was in Washington School [in Oakland, California]. Almost anything that you could do at that time to advance people, say, in the PTA, was supposed to be leading everybody to the left and, eventually, into the Party and, eventually, to a revolution. That was the idea.

Even being in the PTA?

It was the time of Little Rock, and there was a woman called Daisy Bates. The woman who braved the mobs to lead her child into the newly unsegregated school.

There was a front-page story about this heroic mother, and that was the day of the PTA. Being the cookie chairman, I was on the executive board and we had a meeting, so I brought this picture from the newspaper into the PTA and said, "Now, I think this is what the PTA should do—we should pass a resolution commending this brave mother."

The chairman of our PTA said, "Well, our PTA can't do that. That sort of resolution has to be passed by the district. It's not appropriate for our school PTA."

I said, "Well, all right, in that case I'll amend my motion. We should send a memo to the district to pass such a resolution and we should send it to the President of the United States and other people."

My motion died for lack of a second. No one would second it. So I said, "Well, you can stuff your cookies. Good-bye." And that was the end of my time in the PTA.

So it didn't work out in the PTA, but tell me about something you feel you really influenced in your life.

I always think that driving the Famous Writers School bankrupt was probably the only absolutely good thing I can think of. [I wrote an exposé of that school.] That was one good thing.

But, as you can tell by the things I've written about and taken on, they're all kind of peripheral. The undertakers are peripheral. Funerals are peripheral. Funeral directors are peripheral. The funeral industry is peripheral. The birth industry is less so, but some of the reviewers really rather panned the book [*The American Way of Birth*] on the ground that a lot of the things I wrote about had been written before, which was rather true, actually. And again, these things are not the great overriding things that are going to effect all of our lives, like nuclear war for example.

Birth and death?

Birth and death happen, but the kind of funeral that people have, even if they get cruelly overcharged and even if funerals were a great racket, they're not terribly momentous in the lives of people. I think people took to that book because it amused them. It amused me writing it.

Your own family of origin was fascist—Lord and Lady Redesdale. Your sister was in Hitler's inner circle. So, you becoming a Communist and a left-wing activist was very rebellious in your family. But your children have followed in *your* footsteps. You have really raised a new generation of leftists.

I suppose I have. The children were always a part of the work we did with the Civil Rights Congress. That was when we moved to Oakland in 1947, the Civil Rights Congress was the only game in town. And my daughter, Constancia, was with me when I had to go before the California [House Un-American Activities Committee] for being a member of the Communist Party. She is now fifty-four. She was in the South all through the civil rights movement. My oldest grand-child is twenty-eight. A few years ago he said something like "It's not fair. People my age really envy our mothers and fathers and grand-parents for being able to be a part of all of these movements." He was thinking in my case the Spanish Civil War and so on, and in his mother's case of the whole southern civil rights effort. He was think-ing that his own generation was all at loose ends, they didn't have any direction or particular place to go. If there was still a Communist Party, that might give young people more direction, but my grandson is doing good work too. He is a lawyer now, and he's working in the public defender's office in [Washington,] D.C. That's where he wants to be.

Do you still think that there will be a revolution?

I think it's very far in the future now.

I wouldn't like to say that the things we did were illusory. I still think the things we did in my day, and subsequently in my children's day with the civil rights movement, were the things that moved the country along when it was moving along.

But as far as socialism, I can see that it's going to be a long time. I don't know how it's going to come about, but I also can't see how people are going to survive without it. Somehow, I don't know, per-haps somebody will come along with the answers.

Whether there will ever be a Communist revolution or not, we can take what we need from the ideas of socialism, communalism, and basic sharing as we create our own villages and communities. No matter what our family structures or political leanings, we all have to admit that we need each other. Maybe now more than ever.

Chapter 7

"Family Values"

When left, right, and center agree, watch out. They probably don't know what they're talking about. And so it is with "the family" and "family values."
—*Katha Pollitt,* Reasonable Creatures

As I write this, the American welfare system, which was designed in the 1930s to ensure that we all had some very basic necessities for our kids, is being smashed from all sides and, I fear, will be all but history by the time you read this.

As a former welfare mom, I feel like one of the last to get over the bridge before it collapsed. But I'm still optimistic: The revolution is coming. The welfare "reform" of the late 1990s will go down in history as one of the last gasps of the patriarchy. Those boys in Washington will take their misogynist, antifamily legislation one step too far, and unless they've ever seen 10 million mamas fighting for their young, they'll be in for the shock of their sorry lives. Yep. We are going to see an end of the strict-father model in politics as well as in parenting, and we will move into a much more nurturing historical time. But until then we have to deal with the Republicans. And we may even have to explain to our children that just a few short years ago our society didn't toss mothers and children out onto the street. Then some evil politicians came along and started trying to trick people with phrases like "family values." Eventually people started to fall for it, but the change didn't happen overnight.

When I was about seven months pregnant, the Berlin Wall came down. The old Italian veterans I knew cried in the bars and told me that someday my daughter would breathe in a world with no walls at all. Little did they or I know that just as the so-called Soviet threat was being eased in Western minds, a new public enemy was being pumped up to take the number-one slot: me. Unwed teenage welfare moms soon became the ultimate American nightmare. Not that we weren't considered scum all along, but the early 1990s saw a seriously intensified demonization of moms. As soon as the papers were finished reporting "The Breakdown of the Soviet Union," it was on to "The Breakdown of the American Family." To be unwed was bad, to be young was worse, to be on public assistance was, well, practically criminal. But when you listened to the politicians rail on about how we'd caused every societal bummer except maybe freeway gridlock, you noticed that it was the word "mother" they uttered with the most disdain. The details of our motherhood were important, but our main crime seemed to be having children at all, under any circumstances.

"I was sitting around nursing Leron and watching some politician on CNN rant about how single moms are ruining the country, and how

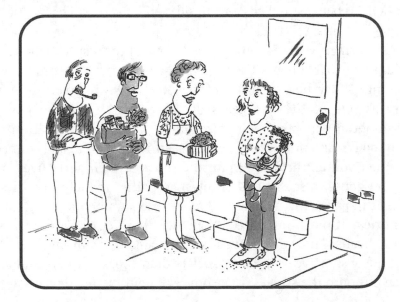

parents aren't paying attention to what their kids watch on TV, and how the American family is such a mess," remembers Tracy, a twenty-one-year-old mother. "And it suddenly occurred to me that this guy was talking about me. About my family. He was basically saying that Leron and I had caused everything from the L.A. riots on down."

Tracy was more than a little shocked to discover that she had become a "political issue." At first she got mad, but as the politician kept talking, he started to sound funny. Hilarious, in fact. "I started busting up," she said. "Imagine. Here I thought I'd been minding my own business, and all of the sudden, Leron and I are dangerous revolutionaries."

My dad, a pretty eccentric guy who lives in Hawaii, recently called and told me that he was writing a paper about all the folks people tend to blame their problems on. You know, Communists, religious groups, people of certain races, and, of course, mom. He said he was having an easy time clearing most of the suspects, but mom, well, that had a certain ring to it. He wasn't at all sure he could write convincingly that all of his problems *weren't* his mom's fault. Now, my dad knows what I do for a living, so I'm going to give him the benefit of the doubt and assume he was sort of playing devil's advocate, but even if *he* was joking, a lot of folks share the sentiment.

Check Your "Family Values" IQ

Politicians and other strange people have been spouting all kinds of nonsense in the name of "family values" over the past few years. So, have you bought the bullshit? This little quiz should help clear things up.

1. The average woman on welfare is
   a. a white teenage mother of three.
   b. a black, never-married woman in her twenties with nine children.
   c. a white, divorced thirty-year-old mother of two.

2. Historically speaking, teen pregnancy did what in the 1990s?

    a. Skyrocketed.

    b. Declined.

    c. Rose to 1970s rates after a slight decline in the 1980s.

3. About what percent of homeless single-mother families are fleeing abusive men?

    a. 25 percent.

    b. 80 percent.

    c. 50 percent.

4. What is the best predictor of how a student will do on his or her SATs?

    a. Gender.

    b. Race.

    c. Family income.

    d. Family structure.

5. The typical teen mom is

    a. a thirteen-year-old woman of color who doesn't want her baby.

    b. a low-income sixteen-year-old prostitute and high school dropout who couldn't figure out how to use the pill.

    c. a low-income eighteen- or nineteen-year-old white woman who wants her baby.

6. All reliable studies show that everything from the crime rate to educational underachievement can be blamed on . . .

    a. out-of-wedlock teen pregnancy.

    b. single motherhood.

    c. the economy, stupid.

7. Feminism is the radical notion that

    a. men suck.

    b. women should practice witchcraft and kill their families.

    c. women are people.

8. Which of these men was raised by a single mom?
   a. Bill Clinton.
   b. Newt Gingrich.
   c. Jesus.

Scoring: Yes, ladies, they are all "c," except number 8, which is a, b, and c. Jesus, as you may recall, was the son of one of the most revered unwed teenage homeless mothers in history.

What's a Girl to Do?

Back in '94, Jennifer Ireland, a then-twenty-year-old single mom, made national headlines when she lost custody of her baby daughter because she planned to put her in day care while attending college. The baby's dad, who had shown no interest in Jen's pregnancy when he was busy with high school football, was suddenly considered ideal by the clueless Michigan judge because he planned to leave baby Maranda with his mother instead. Jen appealed and finally got Maranda back, but talking to this strong mom got a lot of folks thinking: What's a girl to do? "Family values" enthusiasts don't want us to have abortions, they don't want us on welfare, and they don't, apparently, want our kids in day care. So what do they want? Jen certainly couldn't figure it out. "I've done everything to get where I am," she told *Hip Mama* in the middle of her case. Although she was thankful for the support she had gotten from women around the country, even the most well meaning among us were starting to get to her. "I'm put up on a pedestal and I have to be better than everyone, not just better than other teen parents, but better than everyone in the whole world."

With Jen's dilemma in mind, a few friends and I convened a little "family values" caucus. Being objective, rational, and intelligent women, we were sure that with a few pots of coffee we could figure out what we were *supposed* to do if we wanted to please the family values crowd. Here's what we came up with:

DON'T	DO
Have sex	Repent
Masturbate	Repent
Be a lesbian	Repent
Get pregnant	Repent
Get abortions	Put your baby up for adoption and then spend years repenting
Be childless	Repent
Be on welfare	Be independently wealthy
Work	Repent
Put kids in day care	Repent
Drop out of school	Repent
Go to school	Repent
Be single	Get married
Be married to a dork	Pray for the dork
Get divorced	Repent
Be busy	Look busy
Be lazy	Do nothing
Get mad	Repent
Question authority	Thank God you're oppressed because now you'll get into heaven for sure

The Dreaded "Familia Nervosa"

"My son's not a member of a nuclear family, but he plays one on TV," my single dad friend used to tell me. He was talking about a cute little telecommunications commercial that featured his low-income biracial kid who lived with him in a crooked little house on the poor side of the city. In the commercial, the kid played the son of an executive in a suit and a stay-at-home mom who appeared to be the same race.

We all know that if we get our ideas about what a good body looks like from mainstream women's magazines, we are setting ourselves up for low self-esteem and eating disorders. It sometimes takes us a little longer to realize that if we get our ideas about what an ideal family looks like from TV commercials and mainstream parenting magazines, we are setting ourselves up for low family-esteem and perhaps even the dreaded Familia Nervosa—a common disease marked by symptoms of trying to sound chipper when you do housework, going to the beauty parlor and saying "Make me look like Kathie Lee," and attempting to stay married to colossal dorks.

So stop reading the mainstream parenting mags already! And know that when you see a yuppie-cheese-head family on TV, in reality they probably live in a crooked house on the questionable side of town, and they ain't even married. They used the money they got from doing the

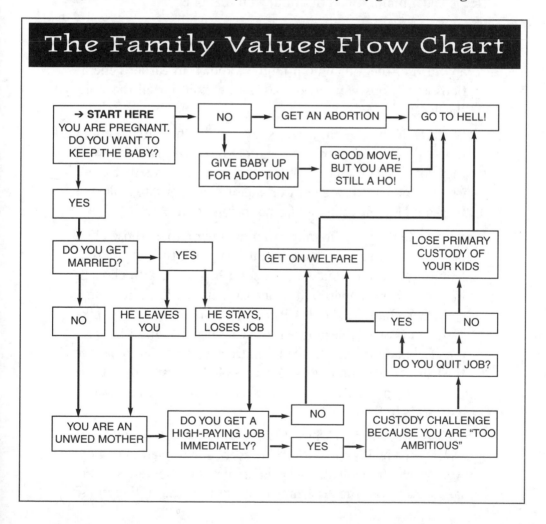

The Family Values Flow Chart

→ **START HERE**
YOU ARE PREGNANT.
DO YOU WANT TO
KEEP THE BABY?

NO → GET AN ABORTION → GO TO HELL!

GIVE BABY UP FOR ADOPTION → GOOD MOVE, BUT YOU ARE STILL A HO!

YES

DO YOU GET MARRIED? → YES

GET ON WELFARE

LOSE PRIMARY CUSTODY OF YOUR KIDS

NO   HE LEAVES YOU   HE STAYS, LOSES JOB   YES   NO

DO YOU QUIT JOB?

YOU ARE AN UNWED MOTHER → DO YOU GET A HIGH-PAYING JOB IMMEDIATELY? → NO

YES → CUSTODY CHALLENGE BECAUSE YOU ARE "TOO AMBITIOUS"

commercial to stay off welfare for two months, and now they are even poorer and more eccentric than you are.

Labels to Make You Feel Bad

Here are a few of the categories you will likely find yourself in after you have kids. While some mamas identify with them, I can pretty much guarantee you that they were all thought up by journalists, politicians, and/or ad wizards who were *not* mamas.

So far in my career as a mom, I have been called every one of these except "older mom." And I'm working on that one.

- •At-Home Mom: Also called Stay-at-Home Mom, this generally refers to married women with children under six. Specifically, any turn-of-the-millennium mother, known in earlier generations as a "housewife" who does not get paid for all the work she does.

- •Working Mom: Literally refers to any mother. In common usage, refers only to working mothers who get paid for work they do outside the home. While the term suggests that those who do not get paid are not working, it is also used to make the Working Mother feel guilty for not being home more.

- •Soccer Mom: While literally meaning any mother whose child plays soccer, this term has come to identify a turn-of-the-millennium "at-home" middle-class suburban mom with elementary school–age children. It is unclear whether it matters what sport her children play (or if they play anything at all). Like "At-Home Mom," this phrase is used at once to make other parents feel bad for missing their children's games and to belittle the work Soccer Mom does. Since her kids are supposed to be part of a team, Soccer Mom drives either a minivan or a wagon with seats in the trunk.

- •Welfare Queen: Also called Welfare Mom, this term was first widely used by President Ronald Reagan, and it referred to a few women who fraudulently received hundreds of thousands of dollars a year from the government. In current usage, the phrase has come to identify any mother who receives more than about five dollars a year through any government program. While this term, if broken down literally, means "preeminent and faring well," it has come to mean, ironically, "Big Loser."

•**Teen Mom:** Literally, any woman under twenty who has children. In common usage, it refers specifically to any unwed mother who had her first child before the age of twenty (even if she is now sixty). Also in common usage, this term is virtually identical to "Welfare Mom," although most people who use the phrases interchangeably know full well that very few teenagers actually receive welfare.

•**Older Mom:** Taken literally, this phrase is totally meaningless as it does not specify whom the Older Mom is older than. However, in common usage this phrase refers to any woman who gives birth after the age of culturally sanctioned maternity. In turn-of-the-millennium America, the window for culturally sanctioned maternity seems to be between the ages of approximately twenty-nine and thirty-two.

•**Bad Mom:** This phrase refers generally to any mother who is not the Virgin Mary. According to those who blame Mary for her son's "martyr complex," however, even she is not exempted from the label.

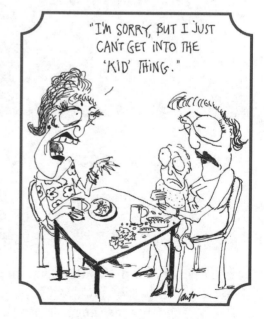

"I'M SORRY, BUT I JUST CAN'T GET INTO THE 'KID' THING."

Talking Back

They Say, eyebrows raised . . .	You Say, smiling . . .
It was so nice when children had mothers *and* fathers.	Yeah, Nazi Germany was full of two-parent families.
You look too young to have a child!	I have a *fabulous* plastic surgeon.
I just don't know *how* you do it.	With your tax dollars.
Are you the nanny?	No, I'm the grandma.
There are so many broken homes . . .	Actually, *my* home is in much better repair than it was when my ex-husband used to put my head through the walls.

Why No One Ever Wins the "Debate"

Mamas sometimes ask me, *But isn't there some way to really talk to these people?* If there is, I certainly haven't found it. And believe me, I've tried. My most comical attempt came back in the summer of 1995 when I agreed to go to Washington, D.C., and be on an MTV panel with Tabitha Soren and a few other twentysomething suckers. Our task was to debate Speaker of the House Newt Gingrich. (Okay, laugh, but it seemed a reasonable proposition at the time.)

"My nephews are so excited that I'm going to be on MTV" were the first words I heard out of Newt's mouth as he headed down the hall toward the studio's green room.

As he walked in, his face was flushed and he seemed like a third-grade teacher coming backstage to greet his students before a school play. "Now are you all ready?" he asked as he moved around the room. "Are we ready?"

Although I'd toyed with the idea of refusing to shake the Speaker's hand when I met him for the first time, instead I took his hand and squeezed it as hard as I could, imagining that I might break his fingers, but he hardly noticed. He was busy describing the T-Rex skull we could see if we came by his office later in the day. "Her name's Rexanne," he said proudly before he was whisked off to the makeup room by an eager production assistant.

"This is surreal," a guy next to me whispered. And believe me, it was.

The show we were about to tape was called "Newt: Raw." And at twenty-five, I was the oldest panelist in the group, which included Jonathan, a conservative painting contractor with greenish hair; Rob, a short Marxist type who worked for *HotWired*; Khakasa, a liberal med student from New York and the only woman of color among us; Jim, a member of Dartmouth's conservative union; and Kate, a tall blond pro-lifer who once worked for Ross Perot. The six of us, along with Tabitha, had spent the entire previous day rehearsing the forum with *Newsweek* columnists sitting in as Newt. If all went as planned, we (well, at least Rob, Khakasa, and I) would kick Newt's butt.

Before I turned to follow the group out of the green room to tape the real thing, an MTV staffer grabbed my shoulder. "Newt's never been publicly confronted by a *real* welfare mother," she said excitedly. "Give him hell."

POLITICAL CORRECTION # 8,525

~~SLEAZEBAG~~

ETHICALLY DAMAGED

As the makeup artists transformed Newt's complexion from light beet to pale peach, the six of us marched out to the set, which consisted of hundreds of yards of velvet and a fake granite table that looked like it belonged on *The Flintstones*.

"Ariel," a columnist from *Newsweek* said, nudging me before we sat down, "I can't wait to hear him try to explain welfare to you. That's what I'm waiting for."

As the tape rolled, Newt was quick to set the tone for the morning. He began by answering a question from Jim with a slow, methodical explanation about the link between liberal student loan policies and the national debt, between liberal student loan policies and economic injustice, between liberal student loan policies and the whole break-down of Western Civilization.

"But Mr. Speaker," Rob tried to interject before he was deftly cut off.

"Let me finish," Newt told him.

"But Mr. Gingrich," Khakasa tried.

"Just wait," he said, flicking his hand as if to shoo her away.

As he continued, there was a collective sigh among panelists that MTV's audio equipment didn't quite pick up. As Newt finished his introductory lecture and we went to the first commercial break, Tabitha had a moment to joke with the him. "Can't we call you Newtie?"

"If you call me Newtie I swear I'll come across the table at you," he snapped with a smile.

"How about Newt Doggie Dog?" Dartmouth's conservative asked.

"Who's your favorite Beatle?" Rob wanted to know. (We had been warned not to ask him such frivolous questions on the air.)

"Ringo, I think." Newtie nodded. "Yes, Ringo."

As we all watched the first package superficially covering the Speaker's life and career that would be spliced into the otherwise unedited show, even the conservative panelists exchanged looks of panic. We expected a hard-hitting look at where the man born as Newton McFearson came from, but the tape looked and sounded more like a video valentine toast to the dude.

As the show continued, panelists challenged various aspects of the "Contract with America" and Newtie calmly explained the bizarre logic behind it all.

I looked around the table and it was as if it suddenly dawned on each of us that we were attempting a political and policy debate with the Samurai of debaters. The research MTV staffers had fed us was shoddy at best, and we sat around the set that morning faced with one simple fact that we had overlooked: Newt is a teacher. One of those very strict old-school teachers. And with Professor Gingrich there is no debate. There is only education. He has the answers. We are ill-pre-pared for the exam.

By the time my two welfare minutes rolled around, the audio equipment easily recorded the resignation in my voice.

"I had my daughter when I was nineteen years old and I was about to start college, and I needed welfare child support in order to go to college," I told Newtie. "My question to you is just what would you have me do in that situation?"

A little of the morning redness returned to his face as he answered me in the slow and methodical lecture tone we had by now grown used to. "We would keep the Women Infants and Children nutrition program, we would keep the food stamp program to enable you to get food. And we would require you to either go to school or to work. Those are the basic requirements, so I doubt if there would be any changes at all."

There was silence at the table for just a moment as the camera focused on my look of total confusion. I wondered if, perhaps, I had misinterpreted all Newtie's plans for welfare. Or perhaps I'd heard him wrong now. In any case, I couldn't believe that the most public "welfare buster" in the United States was sitting less than six feet from me and telling me, with a straight face, that nothing was going to change.

"Actually," I finally said, "under your plan it would only be for two years, so I'd be able to get, like, half a B.A. I wouldn't really be able to go to school."

Newtie cleared his throat and changed his tone slightly. "Okay," he explained as if I were a five-year-old asking for an allowance. "That's right. The question is whether welfare is the way to subsidize education."

When I reminded him that the welfare didn't go to the university but rather subsidized unpaid child support, his tone changed again. His face was flushed, and I thought for sure he was going to tell me that I was a bad student who didn't understand anything. A student who had forgotten her lines.

"The idea that a twelve-, thirteen-, fourteen-year-old is given cash to get pregnant is very destructive," Newtie almost shouted.

Before I had a chance to bring us back to the current question and remind him that I was not twelve, thirteen, or fourteen, Jim interrupted.

"I agree, Mr. Speaker," he said assuredly. "Thirteen-year-olds shouldn't be having children when they are still children themselves."

I was ready to slap someone and Jim was the closest to me. I turned to look at him and he shut up. But Newtie was already running with the new topic. I took a deep breath and tuned into what he was saying. "Twelve-, thirteen-, fourteen-year-old drug addicts, prostitutes, in the inner city . . ." Even Jim looked confused.

"The males need to take responsibility," Newtie was shouting as Tabitha interrupted him to give me the floor back.

"I totally agree that the fathers should pay their child support, but what happens," I said, attempting, for some reason, to sound cordial, "is that when he doesn't pay, I am punished."

"The child is punished," Khakasa corrected.

"Yes," Newtie finally agreed. "The burden should be on the father to pay and not on the mother to collect."

"So you're for guaranteeing that child support?" I asked.

"Yes, uh."

"In the form of welfare?"

"No."

My two minutes were over, and I had accomplished little more than making Newtie a little nervous for about twenty-five seconds.

Kate was anxiously awaiting her turn to ask the Speaker to explain the benefits of corporations to young people who didn't understand how great they were.

"Surreal," I heard someone whisper while the camera was on Kate.

In a few minutes, "Newt: Raw" was winding up.

"My nephews Mark and John will be happy now," Newtie said on the air as if he had promised them a mention. The lights dimmed, and the dozens of TV, radio, and print reporters who had been watching from a back room rushed in, asked a dozen stupid questions, and rushed out again. Newtie was out of the studio in time to open the House, and I headed back through Dulles, through San Francisco, and to Oakland in time to pick up my food stamps and relieve my baby-sitter, all the while wondering how on earth I failed to kick the Speaker's butt.

Obviously, my debating skills weren't what they might have been, but my real mistake, I realized after banging my head against the wall repeatedly for about a week, was that I tried to *talk* to this guy. You can't debate someone who doesn't tell the truth, and, more important, you can't debate someone who is coming at you from a *totally* different worldview.

As cognitive linguist George Lakoff has broken it down for us in his book *Moral Politics: What Conservatives Know that Liberals Don't*, there are those of us who believe in nurturance—those of us, mostly of the liberal persuasion, who pick a baby up when it cries at night—and then there are those of them who believe in the strict-father/strict-teacher/strict-government thang—those, mostly of the conservative persuasion, who think that baby will learn something if they just let it cry and cry and cry. Because most of us think of the government as being, basically, some kind of parental figure, we extend our philosophy of parenting into our politics. As Lakoff told an interviewer for the *East Bay Express*, "Why would Newt Gingrich come up with the idea of taking children away from welfare mothers, putting them in orphanages—especially when it was reported that it would cost much more than paying the welfare mothers to raise them? The reason, of course, is that welfare mothers don't have strict-father morality, but the orphanages do."

But there's also a little something liberals know that conservatives don't. As studies of attachment parenting have all shown, babies who get the attention they need—babies who generally get picked up when they cry—actually become more independent. Babies who are raised with the whole "Cry it out, you'll get over it" theory don't get over it. They just crave *more* attention.

My point is that you can talk to people who are of two minds about the whole "family values debate," and you might have an impact. But the ultra-conservative strict-father types are a different story. They just might be hopeless.

Apocalypse Parenting

I love teaching my daughter about politics. I take her to protests, help her interpret the daily news, and try to teach her everything I can about the history and current possibility of social change.

But as a girl who grew up watching movies like *The Day After* and listening to Dr. Helen Caldicott tapes in the backseat of my parents' car, I'm careful not to scare my kid. The movies were all about the dreaded nuclear holocaust. And Caldicott was this radical Australian babe who spoke out about the Cold War and advocated a nuclear freeze. "The planet is terminally ill," she would proclaim on her tapes, and I remember being convinced that I would never see my eighteenth birthday. She was a doctor. And she had pronounced the world terminally ill. A lot has been written about this, and there have been more than a few generations who grew up with the same fears as I did—think David Bowie . . . "we've got five years . . ."

Dr. Caldicott told her listeners to assure us kids that our parents were doing something about the nuclear threat and that we should feel optimistic. But we didn't feel optimistic. To say we worried might just be the understatement of the century. We got all bent out of shape and rushed around through our teenage years with even more urgency than those adolescent hormones require.

Politicize Those Babies

- Take your children to political events and protests. (Feel free to leave when the riot cops get there.)

- Take your children to the polls and show them the voting process.

- Teach your kids about the history of social change movements.

- Make a career switch or pursue an education in a field you can be radical in (like P.R. for progressive companies, political work, advocacy, etc.).

- Teach your children about boycotts and observe them.

- Make sure there is a steady and diverse stream of radical women and men in your children's lives.

- Make a project out of sending obnoxious faxes to obnoxious politicians. This will teach them how to use technology too! My favorite obnoxious fax to date is shown on page 151. I sent it soon after my local loser governor out here in California accused welfare mothers of "promiscuousness" and "idleness."

Indeed, you can politicize children into virtual manic-depression.

When Maia was a preschooler and we started seeing all this kid-oriented stuff about saving the world by planting trees and recycling cans into weird parade floats, I started experiencing a little déjà vu. I mean, what is up with bringing a kid into the world and immediately telling her it's her job to save it?

Aren't there ways to teach our kids about environmentalism, peace-making, and whatever else we want them to know without scaring the training pants off of them? I think there are.

FAX TO CALIFORNIA GOVERNOR PETE "PROMISCUOUS AND IDLE WELFARE MOTHERS" WILSON: (916) 445-4633 OR SEND TO THE OFFICE OF THE GOVERNOR, STATE CAPITOL BUILDING, SACRAMENTO, CA 95814

WE MAY BE PROMISCUOUS, BE WE AIN'T IDLE!

We Are Mothers,
We Are Strong,
Don't Keep Doing
Our Children Wrong

MISOGYNY: LOOK IT UP, STAMP IT OUT!

HAPPY VALENTINE'S DAY, PETE . . . THIS YEAR WE ASK THAT YOU LOOK WITHIN YOUR HEART: ARE YOUR ACTIONS BASED ON MISOGYNY? RACE HATRED? GREED? DO YOU THINK YOUR CHILDREN ARE MORE IMPORTANT THAN OURS? LISTEN WITH YOUR HEART. (AND REPENT, LOSER!) YOU ARE KILLING CHILDREN AND ABUSING FAMILIES! ONLY YOU CAN STOP THE WAR ON MOTHERS AND CHILDREN!

War sucks because people get hurt and die; we should not take part in war. Environmentalism and recycling are good ways to keep the planet nice. When we plant seeds, cool things grow.

If the world ends next month, we might end up feeling like we lied to our kids—feeding them optimism when the End Was Nigh—but chances are, we are all going to survive our life experiences. I wish someone would have warned me about *that* when I was a kid.

If Yo Mama Were President

So you're tired of white guys in ugly suits running the country? Well, if Yo Mama were president, she'd revolutionize government from top to bottom. What's her platform?

- A meaningful job and minimum income for everyone. Or stay home if you want; Yo Mama will guarantee you livable child support for raising happy, healthy kids.

- Minimum wage? Who cares? What we really need is a maximum wage to solve the lazy-rich-people/high-cost-of-living problem.

- Gays in the military? Sorry. Yo Mama will abolish the military. The Pentagon's budget will be reallocated toward Universal Health Care, Universal Child Care, quality public education, and guaranteeing the absolute right to food, shelter, clean air and water, and good pizza and ice cream in every town.

- What for the ultra-conservatives? you ask. Yo Mama will offer free passage into the burning depths of hell for all Right-Wing Dittoheads. She'll even throw a prayer breakfast going-away party.

- Worried about the future of safe, legal abortion? Fear not, Yo Mama promises free abortion on demand. She knows what's up: She has no business in your uterus.

- And Yo Mama's response to domestic violence? This president will never ask "Why doesn't she leave?" She'll make *him* leave. There will only be two options for batterers: graduate from an approved overcoming violence program or be exiled into hell with the Dittoheads, where both will be haunted by volunteer welfare queens and the ghosts of dead social policy victims.

• Had it with ridiculous family court decisions? Family issues and decisions on child custody will be taken out of the courts and given to a council of our feminist grandmothers.

And this is just the beginning.

Yo Mama sounds like a crazy Commie, you say? Perhaps she is and perhaps she isn't. She's a mama, and she won't stand by and watch her children starve while the politicians in Washington sound something like the invisible grown-ups in *Peanuts* . . . "Wha-wha-wha, wha-wha-wha . . ."

Wondering how she'll accomplish all of this? Then you're being too damn *practical*, girls. And anyway, rumor has it Yo Mama has something no other politician can lay claim to: a functioning brain and a magic wand. Read her hips: She's from a place called Reality; she'll end patriarchy as we know it, offer tax breaks to all radical fringe activists, and guarantee a tasty tofu stir-fry in every pot.

~~~~~~~~~~~~~~~~~~~

Rebel Mom

What Social Science Really Tells Us

Judith Stacey, mama of one, professor of sociology and gender studies, author of In the Name of the Family: Rethinking Family Values in a Postmodern Age

How did you get involved in the "family values" debate?

I was drawn into the debate with [my research on divorce for my book *Brave New Families*]. One of the surprising things I found when I was doing that research was the role that divorce plays in the building of family ties. Everyone sees it as this rupture, and it certainly is very serious, but divorce also provides an opportunity to expand family relations. With remarriages it ends up numerically expanding the number of kinship ties. Sometimes it also ends up expanding the resources available, when there are two homes.

Tell me about your research on the "family values" campaign itself. . . . In your book you say there has been an orchestrated right-wing campaign to convince President Clinton, the media, and many Americans that two-parent families are superior to other family structures.

When I started looking around, there was actually an organized and well-funded campaign, and social scientists were involved in it. It was an attempt to move the Democratic Party to the center and it is tied to a host of initiatives—the assault on single mothers, the backlash against gay and lesbian families—and it played an ugly role in the repeal of welfare.

If you read history and anthropological research, you will see that families have been incredibly diverse throughout history and certainly are today. Not all children are alike, and the quality of family and kinship relations have so much more to do with child welfare than family structure. I think family structure has almost no effect on child welfare, but even the more mainstream researchers who don't share my politics will say that it has only a very limited effect. And yet the campaign claims that social scientists have a consensus that two-parent families are better. They only use the research they like, when they like it. That is a complete violation of social science principles, and yet they claim to be speaking on behalf of social science.

Can you put the current debate in a historical context for us?

There's no question that there's been a dramatic change in family life over the past two decades. So it's not surprising that people are confused. At the same time, there has been a decline in living wages and a real polarization between the haves and the have-nots.

In periods of rapid change, and especially in times of economic hardship, the number of female-headed households always goes up—it was true in the nineteenth century, it was certainly true in the 1930s, although the rosters didn't always show it because many men resorted to "the poor man's divorce," which was abandonment.

In this case, the family change has been so visible and so widespread that people are ready to believe that what I call "the breakdown of the modern family" causes crime, causes economic hardship, and on down the line. You see, there is this old trick in social science—confusing correlation with causality. When two things happen at once, it's easy to say that one is causing the other, but often there is something else causing them both.

I happen to think that these things are all part of a larger package, that they are not the result of a change in values but have to do with changes in the economy—the decline of the living wage, the decline of labor unions, the exporting of jobs, the globalization of capitalism, the increasing jobs in the service sector, and the decreasing jobs in industry.

If you really wanted to increase the number of people who are married, the easiest way to do that would be to create living-wage jobs, especially for men. This is totally uncontroversial. This is not a mystery.

Can you talk about how you see gay and lesbian families as being on the cutting edge.

I do see them on the cutting edge, although I don't see them as dramatically different from other families.

Once you have divorce as routinized, and you have women's work in the labor force routinized, you are guaranteed a very patchwork kind of family life. You get more single parenthood, you get stepfamilies and blended families with divorce and remarriage, so you've already ensured a lot of family diversity.

But I do see gay and lesbian parents as being on the vanguard, because in order to choose to be a family in a society that doesn't support or encourage you to be, you have to do it much more intentionally. And for same-sex parents, deciding to have a family does require a different procreative strategy, you automatically have a third party, visible or invisible, involved. It's a much more conscious and reflective process. Things can't be taken for granted. Even when the children are the products of heterosexual unions, it requires struggle and reflection to maintain ties and claims to the children.

On a queer E-mail list I get, you see incredible discussion about what is the meaning of marriage? And what are the advantages and disadvantages? These are not issues specific to gays and lesbians, they are basic questions about rethinking marriage for the twenty-first century. They are issues the vast majority of us are involved with, but not always as consciously. They are also on the vanguard of trying to change family law to meet the realities of family life in the twenty-first century.

"The American Family," particularly that notorious white hetero-sexual Christian nuclear capital-F Family, has become such a legend that no one seems to be able to let go of the ludicrous idea that it's the best and only structure in which to raise a kid. Even when a capital-F, Pat Robertson–style Family turns out to be alcoholic, bloated, and dead, there are all these people running around claiming that this idealized "Family" is perfection, is Kingly, the Elvis of families. It all makes you wonder if the ideal ever existed at all.

As we take a real look around, we discover that all kinds of families are working. We discover that in our diversity, we are strong. And in all of our difference, we have a lot more in common than the ad wizards would ever have us imagine. We all know that married parents divorce, single parents remarry, and blended families get together to start the whole thing again. And the soccer mom, it turns out, isn't so far away from the welfare mom. Many of us have been both. Maybe someday our families will be recognized and valued as the liquid and ever-changing communities that they are.

Chapter 8

Work and School in the Land of Motherhood

Someday the world will be set up so that there's day care everywhere and you can put "mom" on your résumé, no questions asked. Until then we just have to make the system accommodate us, no questions answered. —Jenna, thirty-six

It's 8 A.M. Peter gets up and makes himself a cup of coffee, fills four bowls with corn flakes, and sets a carton of milk in the middle of the table before he shouts "Good morning!" into the back room. After some coaching, a five-year-old stumbles into the kitchen and sleepily pours some milk into his bowl, some onto the table, and some onto the floor.

As Peter struggles to get the three school-age kids ready and off to their various classrooms before he has to be at his own morning college class, his wife, Hannah, rolls out of bed to spend the day with their youngest.

Later in the day Peter will come home with his backpack, the couple will pick up the older kids from school, and Hannah will head off to work the swing shift at her full-time job.

Even though Peter and Hannah are outnumbered two to one by their kids, they manage to get through their days with relatively little spilled milk and a certain amount of grace. But don't call them "naturals."

"This is a dance that took a long time to perfect," Hannah admits.
"Perfect?" Peter says.

And they both have to laugh. Or they might cry.

The job title "housewife" may have lost some of its honor in recent decades—not to mention its financial feasibility—but every mom knows that dealing with kids is a full-time job. When we also work or go to school, we don't trade one profession for another, we simply start working a double shift.

Nine to Five

More than half of all American moms with kids under the age of one are in the paid labor force. And many of us work outside the home full time. Whether we return to work after a maternity leave or get a new job after we have kids, employment as a mama takes some serious getting used to.

If you've taken a few month's maternity leave, it's good to keep in pretty regular contact with your employer and coworkers while you are gone. Legally, when you return to work, your employer has to offer you the same salary, the same status, and the same benefits as you had before, but not necessarily the same job. Keeping in contact, you can make sure everyone knows you'll be back, and over the months, you'll be able to talk about how things will be when you return.

If you'd rather work part-time when you return to work, you can also consider job sharing. Depending on your field, this is becoming more and more common. If you know another person in your department who is also interested in job sharing, the best thing to do is get together and make a proposal to your manager.

Many companies, like U.S. Sprint long distance, also offer flex time, or full-time employment opportunities with flexible or modified schedules. If modified hours would help your schedule, find out about the options at your company.

Whether you are returning to work after a maternity leave, reentering the labor force after a long time away, or taking on full-time employment for the first time, ask your employer if you can ease into the job. You might be able to go in for a few half days before your first full day of work.

If you are looking for a new job, network with friends, other new moms, and family to find a mama-friendly workplace. *Working Mother* magazine offers good tips year-round, but their annual "Guide to the Best 100 Companies" is a great place to identify your best bets as far as big companies go. They also list which companies offer on-site child care, a little tidbit you can also get from your local chamber of commerce.

No matter how much research you do, however, finding a good company might take some trial and error. "If I had a dollar for every time I heard the words 'flex time,' I wouldn't have needed their damn job," my friend Maria remembers about the first company she worked for after she had her daughter. "But once I got in there, it was a different story. I ended up getting fired because 'flex time' to me meant that I had to come in at 8:30 instead of 8:00 because that's what time my kid's school started. To them it meant nothing." Maria did her homework again and eventually found another company that was serious about its commitment to working moms.

Once you are back in the labor force, the natural time crunch might be exacerbated by the dorks at work (or elsewhere) who try to make you feel guilty for being away from your kids. As if we didn't think to feel guilty all by ourselves, a lot of folks reinforce our worries by telling us how terrible it is to have our kids in day care. This is all bullshit. Whatever your schedule, you can still spend important, quality time with your kids. As Selma, a forty-year-old single mother, tells me, "The time away from home makes me a better mom when I'm here."

Know Your Rights, Ladies

Discrimination against people with children is alive and well both in the workplace and at colleges and universities used to dealing with single, childless students. So we all need to understand, and believe in, our rights and capabilities. As moms, we deserve to be treated just as well as nonmoms. Perspective employers cannot ask us about our mama status, our marital status, or our sexual preference. They cannot ask us about our child-care plans, if we are pregnant, or what kind of birth control we use. They cannot ask us our age, our children's ages, or any such nonsense. If you are asked an illegal question in an interview, don't answer it. Respond with something like "Does your company have a policy about that?" And the loser who saw fit to break the law will understand that you know your rights.

I Hate My Job!

When I asked my friend Lelia about working full time and being a mom, I sort of expected her to come out with some eloquent quote about struggle and balance and priorities and all of that. Instead she told me, "It sucks. Contrary to popular belief, unless it's your true choice, unless you like your job and you *want* to have the career you have, it just doesn't work."

Now, I have half a degree in economics. I know that only 5 percent of Americans like their jobs and the other 95 percent just have to pay the rent. When I see a statistic about how 53 percent of moms with kids under one are in the labor force, I know it's not really because we want to be. Still, Lelia's response bummed me out. "Now I'll have to write about the downside of being in the paid labor force," I thought. And I didn't want to. The media has done such an extraordinary job dissing women who work for pay (while the government cuts off all aid to those who don't) that I hesitate to add anything at all to the pile of guilt we, as a society, dump at the doorsteps of women who work outside the home. But Lelia is right. Hating your job and feeling like you'd honestly rather be at home sucks. But what can we do? "Generally my generation wouldn't be caught dead working for the man," Ani DiFranco has noted. "And generally I agree with them. Trouble is, you gotta have yourself an alternate plan."

One nine-to-five mom I know saved every penny she could for a year and a half after her daughter was born and then moved the family to Mexico. "We have enough to last us two years," she told me. "What we'll do after that, I have no idea." This mama's job paid reasonably well, so she lived as cheaply as she could and kept her mind focused on those two precious years. She could have spent her savings on some kind of security—a down payment on a house, for example—but security, when you aren't happy, is totally overrated. Not to mention that it's always an illusion.

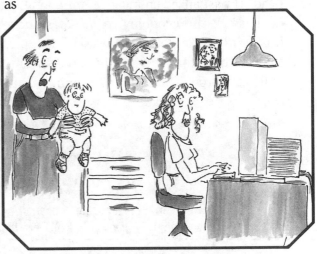

"I think he's downloading."

You probably know what I'm getting at here. Yep. If you hate your job, quit. I know, I know: "Impossible," you say. And maybe it is impossible for you. But then again, maybe you can *make* it possible. Could you work at home? Could you share a place with another family and cut down on your rent? Could you cut your hours—and your day care bill—in half? Could you get yourself fired and live off the unemployment until you figured out what to do next? Could you pool resources with a bunch of other I-hate-my-job girls and open a café? Could you move to Mexico?

A lot of times, after we become mamas, we think we need all kinds of security that we wouldn't have dreamed of when we were single and childless. And it's true that being homeless with kids is a hell of a lot worse than it was without 'em, but sometimes our dreams of white picket fences and bogus symbols of security just make us miserable. And if you never see your white picket fence in the light of day, who's to say it's not green?

Think about your worst-case financial scenario. Would you have to move in with your parents in Florida? Would you be homeless? Or would you just lose your cute red car? Get down to the bare essentials—how much money do you really need? Is there some way to earn it without making yourself miserable? I'm not one of these affluent New Agers who thinks everyone's money problems are in their heads (I "visualized abundance" for a long, long time before I got this book deal); the economy *really does* suck. But sometimes a little imagination can go a long way. I know plenty of mamas who work their butts off for eight or more hours a day basically just to pay their child care providers. Call me a Commie, but that's oppression.

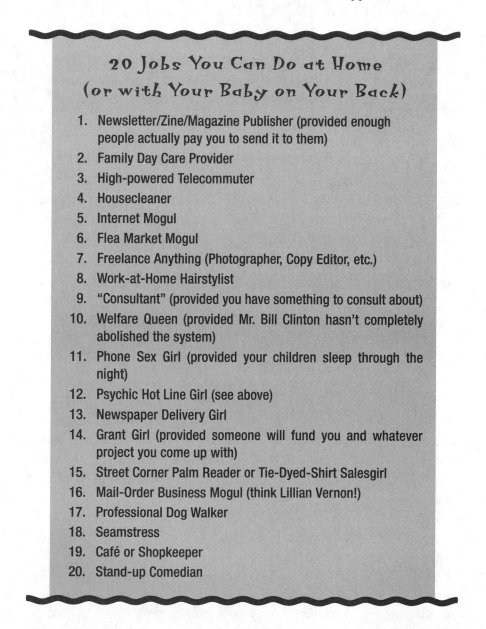

20 Jobs You Can Do at Home (or with Your Baby on Your Back)

1. Newsletter/Zine/Magazine Publisher (provided enough people actually pay you to send it to them)
2. Family Day Care Provider
3. High-powered Telecommuter
4. Housecleaner
5. Internet Mogul
6. Flea Market Mogul
7. Freelance Anything (Photographer, Copy Editor, etc.)
8. Work-at-Home Hairstylist
9. "Consultant" (provided you have something to consult about)
10. Welfare Queen (provided Mr. Bill Clinton hasn't completely abolished the system)
11. Phone Sex Girl (provided your children sleep through the night)
12. Psychic Hot Line Girl (see above)
13. Newspaper Delivery Girl
14. Grant Girl (provided someone will fund you and whatever project you come up with)
15. Street Corner Palm Reader or Tie-Dyed-Shirt Salesgirl
16. Mail-Order Business Mogul (think Lillian Vernon!)
17. Professional Dog Walker
18. Seamstress
19. Café or Shopkeeper
20. Stand-up Comedian

If you hate your job and you don't have savings or family to fall back on, please don't quit right away. Make a plan. Decide you are going to quit in six months or a year. In the meantime, cut down your hours to the bare minimum you need to live on and buy yourself fresh flowers every now and again. Spend whatever time you can figuring out how you will pay the bills when you're out of the rat race, and visualize like hell.

You may decide to start a home business. You could go back to school and borrow money to pay the rent. Two moms I know are working as temp slaves while they write grants (yes, while they are supposed to be doing that temp work) to get funding for a low-income moms' center they plan to start next year. Many combine a bunch of odd jobs to make a living. Not having a real job probably won't end up being any less stressful than whatever you're doing now, but being happy and stressed is a lot more fun than being miserable and stressed.

Back to School with Baby

One night stands out in my memory. It was 10 P.M. My daughter, then four and a half, was in the living room listening to Doc Watson sing *Songs for Little Pickers* as I was desperately trying to concentrate on the beginning of a term paper—due the next day. She should have been in bed by then. I should have started the paper two weeks earlier. But these were the kinds of details I gave up worrying about early in my first year as a single parent/college student.

It all started when Maia was five months old. We were on our way to buy a pink mobile home near the coast. As I was driving along, considering our uncertain future, I remembered, *Wait. I wanted to go to college. Graduate school even.*

I made a U-turn, stood up the real estate agent, and headed for the nearest bookstore to spend part of our trailer down payment on a thick guide to four-year colleges. Almost without realizing it, I had decided to join the estimated 7 to 10 million "nontraditional" students nationwide who decided to go back to school in the 1990s, two thirds of whom were women and many of whom had children, according to a report from the Census Bureau.

At the time I didn't know all I'd have to consider in choosing a school. I didn't think about how much work school would be. I didn't realize quite how much it would cost. (Yes . . . most of the advance I got for this book was immediately claimed by the student loan sharks.) I didn't imagine that I'd be sitting through orientation leaking milk, or writing papers to the tune of "Froggy Went A-Courtin," but even if I had known, I would have made the same decision.

Student parents cite all kinds of reasons for going back to or continuing school after they have kids, but most I've talked to say they wanted to make a better life for themselves and their children, and thought their school schedules could be more flexible than trying to juggle paid work and child rearing. (Read: "It beats pumpin' gas.")

"After I had Rose, school seemed more important," my friend Xena told me when she was a senior in college. "When it was just me I thought I'd try to be a writer, a dancer, or an artist. I could bum around and have funky roommates. But when there was someone else dependent on my income, I decided to go to college."

In choosing a school, we have to consider all the factors traditional students look at, and a hell of a lot more. Public universities are not only less expensive than private ones, but many offer subsidized family housing and day care. "We were counting on me getting into the University of California because they'd give us day care and a place to live," says Winston, a junior in college.

But a lot of folks with kids choose smaller private schools too. "It's a trade-off," one mom says. "When I started as an undergraduate with my first child, I picked a little college because the atmosphere seemed friendly—but then I had to borrow a ton of money."

Smaller schools can also be, shall we say, a little more *flexible* with admission requirements. When I was ready to apply to schools, I had a lot of enthusiasm and a decent essay, but I had never quite finished high school. (I think I passed a total of two semesters.) In my guide to four-year colleges, though, I found a small liberal arts school where I managed to convince the director of admissions to let me in. The college managed to stay afloat for two years—just long enough for me to accumulate the units and grade point average to transfer.

You can also choose the junior-college-for-the-first-two-years route instead. As Winston says, "It's cheap and you can get the admissions requirements for the four-year school taken care of."

No matter which way we go, there is the question of tuition—not to mention child care, keeping roofs over our heads, and eating every once in while. Unfortunately, most financial aid is earmarked for full-time students, so going to school part-time often ends up being more difficult than going full time, which you can fund with loans, grants, work-study programs, scholarships, family contributions, and government resources like welfare.

In my six years back at school, I think I averaged about four hours of sleep each night, found myself nursing an infant during an economics final, and turned in many a paper with scribbles in the margins. And although I often thought wistfully of my pink trailer near the coast and a morning shift at the corner store, I ended up being able to spend a lot more time with my daughter during her preschool years than I could have with full-time work.

On that night I sat writing my term paper to *Songs for Little Pickers*, my daughter fell asleep on the living room floor. She opened her eyes for a moment as I carried her to the bedroom and changed her into her pajamas. Feeling bad about letting her fall asleep on the floor without her usual bedtime story, I asked if she thought I should quit school—if she would like it if I never went to class and we ate really good dinners and took time to walk (not drive) to the park. Before letting her eyes fall closed again, she asked, "And then do what? College is fun."

False Starts

Beware! An army of con artists sustains itself with mama desperation.

I was still in school when I first tried to do the working-mama thing. I had an infant daughter and a full load of college classes, but I still hoped I could pay the electricity bill somehow. Encouraged by the

Start →	Land Fast-Track Job at New Ad Agency	Maternity Leave (Lose a Turn)	Refuse to Do Vodka Ads Aimed at Pre-schoolers (Roll Again)	Write a Novel (Lose two turns)
Run Away with the Circus!				Decide to Open Home Day Care (Go Ahead 3 Spaces)
Purple Scribbles on Résumé (Go Back 3 Spaces)		*The Real Mommy Track*		Baby Spits Up on Cover Letter (Lose a Turn)
Baby Pours Soapy Water into Business Phone (Roll Again)				Sign Up for Midwifery Classes (Lose $1,500)
Leak Breastmilk on Customers at Table #3 (Lose a Turn)				Oops... Forget to Get a License (Go Back 2 Spaces)
Land Fast-Track Waitressing Job at Café (Go Ahead 1 Space)	Go to Medical School (Lose $75,000)	Open Consulting Business from Home (Go Ahead 4 Spaces)	Baby Gets Sick (Lose a Turn)	Get Pregnant Again (Go Back to Start)

"Work at Home" section of the want ads, I sent off a self-addressed stamped envelope to one of those ads that begins "Earn money stuffing envelopes." For those unfamiliar with this particular con, what you get back in your self-addressed stamped envelope is a longer version of the original ad that promises a job and ends with a request for a nine-dollar "processing and supplies" fee. Being curious as well as desperate, I sent off the nine bucks and got back another flyer. "You see," it read. "You sent me $9 and all I did was stuff envelopes. Put a similar ad in your local paper and see how much money you can make."

Similar work-at-home cons pass themselves off with lines like "Earn money reading books" (you end up with a $30 book *about* earning money reading books), "You deserve freedom of lifestyle" (pyramid scheme!), or some other such nonsense. I know mamas who have lost several hundred dollars on these things.

Swearing off the want ads for a while, I turned to college work-study in hopes of earning some extra cash. Work-study was, after all, on the up and up. My string of jobs ranged from calling prospective students and gushing about my school to teaching statistics on Sunday afternoons. And these jobs seemed good. I earned about $6 an hour and got to wear jeans. What it took me a while to realize, however, was that each dollar I earned in work-study reduced my loan eligibility. Sure, I'd owe a little less when I got out, but my paychecks went straight toward my tuition, leaving my electricity bill sitting unpaid on my kitchen table. Interestingly, social services felt rather possessive when it came to my little work-study check too. For each dollar I earned, I lost a dollar in food stamps. After child care, I was actually *paying* about $3.50 an hour for the privilege of working.

So, like I said: Beware, mamas! If you work, *they* are supposed to pay *you*. Period. Beware of "initial investments." Beware of anything that sounds remotely like "Earn money doing nothing." Beware of "employers" who act like they are trying to sell you a job. Beware of pyramid schemes. Beware of wages that anyone else can claim. Any real employer will let you think about an offer for twenty-four hours. Go home. Do the math. And know what you are getting into.

Check Out Your Potential
Child Care Provider

- Do you like them?
- If it's a day care center, is there at least one teacher for every four or five kids? Do you like all the teachers?
- Do the other kids look happy?
- Is the place clean, well lighted, and someplace you wouldn't mind spending the day?
- Does your kid seem to connect with the care provider?
- Does the provider seem responsive to both your concerns and your kid?
- Will the provider talk to you about how your kid is doing on a regular basis?
- If it's just one person, will it ruin your life if she or he gets sick?
- Does everybody there know CPR? Are first-aid supplies available?
- Are you going to feel weird about leaving your kid with these folks?
- What religious or patriotic beliefs do they plan to pass on to your kid?
- What's the deal with holidays?
- Can you drop in at any time without calling to warn them?
- Does the care provider or do all the teachers at the center look happy and awake?
- Do they have a license? If they aren't required to have one, have you checked their references?
- What's the food situation?
- What hours are child care available?
- If your schedule is not fixed, is that cool with the care provider?
- If you're nursing and expressing milk, does the care provider get a grossed-out look on her face when you say so?
- How do they deal with tantrums and other "behavioral issues"?
- What does the caregiver think of your parenting philosophies?
- Will Rush Limbaugh *ever* be on?

- How much experience does the caregiver have and, if it's a center, how long has it been in operation?
- How much experience does the caregiver have with kids the same age as yours? If it's a day care center, are there age-appropriate toys?
- What happens if your kid gets sick or hurt?
- Do they have a phone they can use to call you if something happens?
- Say, what's the price tag on this whole deal?
- Does the care provider make you feel like a big loser for asking all these questions?
- Trust your intuition, trust your intuition, trust your intuition.

Rebel Mom

Piercing, Transmissions, and Caffeine
Wendy DeJong, tatooed and fancy-shoed mama of one

You work full time now. How soon after Ezekiel was born did you start doing that?

I didn't start working full time until he was three and a half. It was very important to me to stay at home with him, so I worked part-time as a body piercer. Then I borrowed some money and opened a tattoo and piercing shop. I worked by appointment only and my family took care of him.

When I realized I was going to be supporting my family by myself, I had a choice. I could work full time, or I could work part-time and have no money. I decided to work part-time and take that extra time with Ezekiel.

Then what happened?

I decided to move to California, so I had to save up some money. The highest-paying job I could get in the town where we lived was re-building transmissions. That was cool. And it was the first time Ezekiel was in preschool full time. He was three and a half.

Were you worried about putting him in day care?

I worried about it because I was still under the illusion that I was going to have control over what he was exposed to in his life. There were a lot of things I didn't want him exposed to: Power Rangers, Christianity, and the whole concept of shame. But I realized early on that that was something I would just have to deal with.

I was aware that the best hours of my day would be spent with other people. When I got home I was not going to have a lot of energy to throw a hula hoop or sit down on the floor to play.

Also, since I've been working full time, it's easy to fall behind and not cook healthy foods. So I make sure that there is a lot of rice and frozen vegetables in the house, because if there isn't a better plan, I can always make some rice and vegetables and cut up some baked tofu. That's good. But sometimes we go to fast-food places or order pizza too.

How did you find good day care?

Adequate child care is a big issue. It took me a long time to find a place I could afford where I felt comfortable leaving him for the majority of the day. I screened a lot of day care centers over the phone, and often I could tell about them right away. If they seemed like they didn't really have time to talk to me, I crossed them off my list. A cou-ple of centers' big claim to fame was "When your child leaves here he will know how to say the Pledge of Allegiance," so I crossed those places off the list too. Another place was just too far away. Anyway, I narrowed it down to three centers, and then went and looked at them. Finally we lucked into this place that had an opening. The staff was really positive, and it wasn't a rigid structure, it was child-led learning and playing. And, miraculously, I could afford it.

I didn't want Ezekiel to be exposed to any kind of prayer in school or even any talk about the scary aspects of Christianity. The cool thing about the school he's in now is that they talk about and celebrate a wide variety of traditions and holidays. On Chinese New Year they had the good luck pennies and tangerines, for example.

How do you deal with how tired you are at the end of the day?

I try to get Ezekiel to sit down with me and read a book. It gives him a chance to settle down and me a chance to get off my feet—I work at an espresso bar all day now.

Also, at four and a half, he's getting to the age where he's more interested in playing with his friends than playing with me. I have weekends off, so that makes a big difference.

It's nice to be at work and interact with adults. But I'll feel better about working full time when I feel like I am doing something to serve humanity. Not that making coffee isn't helpful, but I have grander aspirations.

Do you think about going into business for yourself again?

I was a piercer for long enough. But I hope to be in a situation where I am working on my own again soon. I want to work with women in the childbirth process, and that will also give me more time with Ezekiel on a day-to-day basis.

A s we are bumping along through the first few years of motherhood—navigating the world of work, school, and child care; learning to fight racism and sexism, isolation, and screaming fits; and balancing our lives so we can spend time with our kids—most women I know become familiar with "the chaos theory of parenting." What exactly is the chaos theory of parenting? It is a growing understanding that, try as we might to find some order and predictability in it all, our lives bring us the random, the weird, the totally and completely unexpected. Just as we think we're getting the hang of one "stage" or another, all of the rules change without warning.

How do we deal with mothering in total chaos? We treat our kids with respect, we listen to them, we parent them thoughtfully, we try to stay open to change, and, when all else fails, we wing it: Parenting has never been an exact science.

PART THREE:

MAJOR BUMMERS

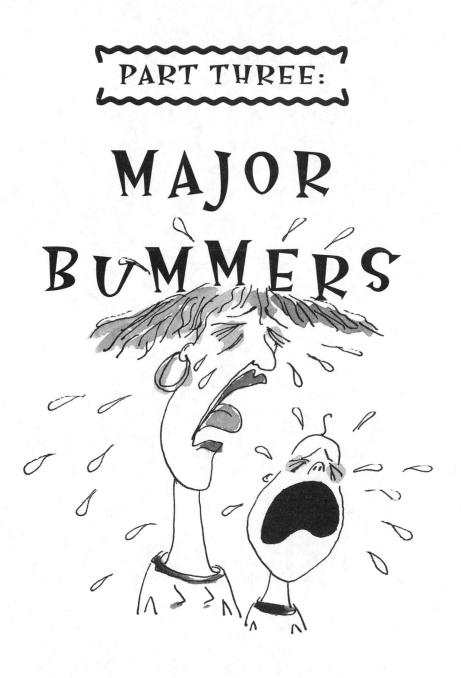

Chapter 9

Nervous Breakdowns
(Are Usually Temporary)

My life is just a sick, sick test. —Julie, twenty-six

I t's like this: I'm taking a full load of classes and working thirty-five hours a week, publishing a zine, trying to make sure there's breakfast on the table every morning, and keeping some handle on the laundry so my daughter's clothes are at least presentable, and my calendar looks like Martha Stewart's (although my hair definitely doesn't). And then, out of the blue, the kindergarten teachers go on strike, or my daughter starts throwing up, or someone tells me that I'm a bad mom and I freeze. I try to take normal breaths, but it's hopeless. I feel like I'm about to burst into tears, and I'm gasping for air like a drowning surfer.

Or it's like this: I've been home with my daughter and a couple of her friends all day. They've gone through all the clean dishes and everything in the house is sticky, and the phone rings and on my way to get it I trip over a robot that starts saying "search and destroy, search and destroy, search and destroy," and when I finally answer the phone it's some very high-maintenance friend without kids calling because she's "bored," and then some kid unplugs the phone right before they all start screaming about whose turn it is to yell commands at the dreaded robot and when they can go home, and all of the sudden I'm screaming and flailing around like I'm possessed by the ghost of Miss Hannigan, the evil orphan keeper.

Now, these episodes are not really nervous breakdowns. That's because (a) they are more like panic attacks, and (b) there isn't any such thing as a nervous breakdown, according to psychiatrists. If we are going to use the proper terminology, then what we commonly refer to as a "nervous breakdown," or simply "Nervous" with a capital N, can be a panic attack, an anxiety disorder, a manic episode, decompensation ("when you just lose your marbles and all your coping mechanisms fly out the window," according to my psychologist friend), depression, or something along those lines. But whatever we want to call the mental or mental/physical conditions that seriously impair our ability to function as moms, as employees, or as partners, they're hell.

Our responses to stress may seem serious or minor, but "losing it" is a normal reaction to life with kids, so we have to watch out. And when we start to fall into that dreaded Nervous abyss, we have to do some damage control.

"What Is Happening to Me?"

Unless you're suffering from paranoia, you know full well that I have no idea what's happening to you. But some very common mama breaks take the form of panic, mania, and depression. As usual, I'm going to give you good research-backed information, but your therapist (we'll get you one over the next few pages if you don't have one) has a degree in this stuff, knows you, and is really the only one who has any business diagnosing you. Having said that, let's see what we're dealing with.

Panic Attack Mom

A panic attack comes on suddenly and peaks after about ten minutes. They are unpleasant, so please don't confuse the diagnostic criteria here with an orgasm. We're looking at four or more of the following symptoms for a bona fide, American Psychiatric Association–endorsed panic attack:

1. Your heart's a-poundin' faster than usual.
2. You're sweating.
3. You're trembling or shaking.
4. You're short of breath.
5. You feel like you're choking.
6. You've got chest pain.
7. You feel like you're going to hurl.
8. You are dizzy, faint, or light-headed.
9. You feel like you're detached from yourself or out of your body.
10. You're afraid you're going to lose control or go crazy.
11. You're afraid you're going to drop dead.
12. You feel numb or tingly.
13. You've got chills or hot flashes.

If you have a panic attack, sit or lie down and focus on your breathing. You are probably not going to die. Call 911 if you need to, but mostly just try to listen to your body and relax. A friend once had a panic attack at my kitchen table and, naturally, started freaking out even more with thoughts of "Omigahd, I'm going to die." Not realizing that she *wasn't* going to die, I fell right into the frenzy, neither of us could calm down, and we ended up spending the night in the emergency room. Obviously it would suck if you really were having a heart attack and you mistook it for a panic attack, but either way, breathing and relaxing will do you a lot more good than fueling your panic with even more fear and loathing.

Manic Mom

A manic episode can be fun at first, but anyone who has ever experienced one in its full technicolor horror knows that after the initial glee, it's anything but fun. Basically, an episode of the manic variety lasts at least a week, but even if you're only on day one, my advice remains, "Talk to a professional, darling!" We're looking for three out of the following seven symptoms, but anything that feels like you're on cocaine when you're not or anything else that seriously disrupts your ability to function deserves attention. (If there's no glee at all, we

might be dealing with agitated depression, but, like I said, if whatever it is impairs you, seek help.)

1. You feel more like you're the queen of the world than usual.
2. You have a decreased need for sleep ("Three hours and I feel *greeaat*!).
3. You talk and talk and talk and talk.
4. Your thoughts are racing.
5. You are easily distractible.
6. You are jamming on all your work and goal-directed activities.
7. You suddenly go on a whirlwind shopping or gambling spree, have sex with ten people (or with the same goofball a dozen times a day), or start investing all kinds of money you don't have in the comeback of the Pet Rock.

Manic episodes usually don't end up requiring hospitalization, but watch out, and try to hang out with people who will stop you if you get out of control. You can do a lot of damage to your life in one short week—even in five short minutes—when you're in a manic state, and the impending crash can be *very* ugly.

Depressed Mom

Depression sucks big time. If your depression lasts more than about three days, please, please, please seek professional help. Depression is a deep feeling of sadness or numbness. For what they call a "major depressive episode," we're looking at a two-week depressed mood or loss of interest or pleasure that also includes five or more of the following symptoms, and it isn't bereavement or some kind of drug-induced thing:

1. You feel tearful, sad, and/or empty most of every day.
2. You're no longer interested, or you no longer find pleasure, in the stuff that used to make you feel good.
3. You're gaining or losing a lot of weight without trying to.

4. You have trouble sleeping or you sleep all of the time.
5. Other folks notice that you seem slowed down and bummed out.
6. You always feel tired and zapped of energy.
7. You feel worthless or guilty.
8. You are having trouble thinking, concentrating, and generally dealing.
9. You have recurring thoughts about death and/or suicide.

This last symptom is particularly heinous for moms. As one depression-experienced mama tells me, "You feel like killing yourself, and then you think of your kids without a mom, and then you would have to kill them too. Aside from the obvious fact that all of this is a seriously bad idea, you know you could never pull it off. What if you killed one kid and the trauma of it shocked you into reality and you couldn't kill yourself?" If this line of thinking sounds remotely familiar, please put this book down and call your local suicide prevention hot line.

And if any of the other symptoms just listed are happening with any kind of frequency, please take it seriously. Denial, in these situations, just doesn't work.

While we're talking about diagnoses, may I say a word about treatment? Medication, while sometimes necessary, is totally overused. I mean, if you've got schizophrenia, bipolar disorder, or some other big-time chemical or chronic thing going on, you have to take your meds, but if you are experiencing unpleasant emotions that you would simply rather not deal with, Prozac just ain't the answer. One mama I know was actually told by a psychiatrist that she had a choice—get into therapy and deal with her problems or, if she didn't think she had time for that, "just take Prozac." In her case, this was utterly ridiculous.

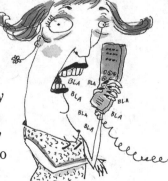

SOME DAYS I JUST HAVE TO TALK ON THE PHONE ALL DAY, even though there's nobody on the other end.

As Clarissa Pinkola Estés notes, "You cannot heal what you cannot feel." And many medications just block our feelings. So watch out for the med-happy doctors, and see if you can't just find a safe place to feel, and to heal.

Some Cool Things About Nervous Breakdowns

- If people find out, they will probably be much kinder and gentler to you in the future.
- Historically, you are in excellent company. Most of the great artists were complete nut cases. (Please try to refrain from following any farther in their footsteps, however. It's no longer stylish to kill yourself or cut off your ear.)
- Foils your inner workaholic.
- Makes for good memoirs.
- Studies have found a significant connection between madness and genius.
- Good excuse not to comb your hair.
- It becomes socially acceptable to yell epithets at yuppie chowderheads when the inspiration hits you.

Getting Help

"My problem when I'm starting to get really overstressed is that I start doing things that actually cause me more stress," says Winona, a thirty-one-year-old mother. "I was already at my limit and then there were all these news stories one month about moms killing their kids and I started freaking, like, am I going to do that? So I took all my kids and went to stay with my aunt and uncle. I somehow forgot that I don't get along with my aunt and uncle at all. I mean, going there was just about the most self-hateful and stressful thing I could have done—and yet there I was, on their doorstep, expecting the visit to help."

Susan, a twenty-four-year-old mom, can relate. "I was pregnant and my toddler son had just been diagnosed with epilepsy. We were in a total financial mess, so what did I do? I stopped going to therapy. I stopped doing all the little things that were keeping me sane and I just stayed home freaking out about my son and thinking, Why am I pregnant again? Why am I going to do this again? So, of course, the whole thing snowballed. When I finally went back to my therapist—I guess it was a month or two later—she sent me to the hospital. Psych ward."

Most of us can feel it when we're nearing the end of our ropes, but often the stuff we start scratching off our calendars are the very things we need—we cancel the therapy, we cancel the support groups, we start looking for help in the places we know we won't find it. In hindsight, our mistakes can look stupid, but in reality, often the first thing to go when we're "losing it" is our ability to reason and our ability to look out for ourselves. If the first thing that pops into our heads is homicide-suicide, most of us can realize that we need to talk to someone else. Fast. But even if our plans aren't life-threatening, we need to seek some guidance. A therapist is great, as long as she's not the kind who just stares at you and nods. But another mom, a trusted friend, a relative who has not failed you in the past—these are good people to call too. If you are fortunate enough to have more than one wise helper in your life, call them all.

I JUST WANT ANOTHER BABY, NOT ANOTHER LITTLE PERSON.

If you don't have a therapist yet, get one. Even if it's only to get out of the house for an hour a week, therapy can be well worth the trouble. These days, most communities have sliding-scale or low-cost counselors, or if your problems can be framed as being work-related, you may even be able to get your employer to pick up the tab. If you can't think of anyone who could give you a good referral, try a counseling referral service, which you can find in the Yellow Pages under "Mental Health Services," "Social Service Organizations," or "Crisis Intervention Services." You can also try the National Mental Health Association at (703) 684-7722.

I realize that I'm telling you to make a lot of phone calls here, so I should mention that I also realize that there are two kinds of people in the world: those of us who don't feel weird about calling for help, and those of us who get so embarrassed and "I can handle it" that we wait until we've got a razor blade in our hand before we ask anyone to intervene. This latter strategy is totally counterproductive. If you're hoping no one will know that you are a nervous/psychotic wreck, waiting until you're about to off yourself really isn't going to help your image. So, please, just try to put your embarrassment and all of that other self-judging crap aside for a few moments. If you absolutely cannot call anyone you know, hot lines really *are* anonymous, and believe me, these folks have heard *it all*.

Take a Deep Breath: Quick Strategies for Damage Control

- Remove yourself from your children: Go in the bathroom to breathe, scream, cry, or whatever.

- Call a hot line.

- Call a friend to come watch your kids.

- If you don't know anyone who can watch your kids, look in the Yellow Pages under "Crisis Intervention Services" to get some respite care.

- Lay down and breathe. Let yourself feel whatever you are feeling. If this gets so intense it starts to scare you, try to think of a more peaceful time and repeat after my therapist: "I give thanks for help unknown already on the way. . . ."

- Take a nap. As you are falling asleep, tell yourself that you will wake up knowing what to do about the situation.

- Call your therapist and leave a long, incoherent message on her voice mail.

- Take a shower and wail about everything that has ever made you sad.

- Draw a picture of all your ooey emotions.

- Make depression dolls, courage masks, and other art thangs

Art and Psyche

Making dolls and other artistic things can be relaxing, inspiring, and cleansing. At first the suggestion might sound somewhat ridiculous—like "just go do some finger painting, honey." But the connection between creativity and madness that has been well documented is so strong because when we get down to our artistic selves, we find a direct line to our subconscious. Don't worry about making things "pretty" here. We're talking about getting your deepest darkest out of your system.

You can make a monkey-puke-green doll that's threaded all wrong, or you can create a gorgeous cocoa-colored doll with sunshine in her hair to represent happier times to come. You can make pretend voodoo dolls of your exes, rag dolls from scraps of too-small kid clothes, or whatever.

If dolls aren't your thing, Luisah Teish, a priestess of Oshun in the Yoruba Lucumi tradition who wrote *Jambalaya*, suggests making a "Mask Macabre" in your fit of depression. This isn't really an activity to do with the kids, so get a baby-sitter. Then sit quietly, frown, and contort your face muscles to get into your pain. Draw how you feel on a paper plate, punch holes in the sides, and tie it to the back of your head. Then scream out all the negative shit until you feel like it's outta there. Throw the mask in the fireplace or into a metal bowl and watch it burn. Then go to the mirror and smile. You are a glorious, strong mama.

And Now a Word from New Age White-Light Girl

I'm no good at channeling. I usually find people who say things like "You create your own reality" annoying, if not downright offensive. I have never felt that I was "one with lettuce." But I am a Californian, so as you've probably already noticed in these pages, there is something of the New Age White-Light Girl in me.

About a year before I started working on this book, the idea of meditating every day started, shall we say, stalking me. When I was a teenager I used to hang out at this Zen Buddhist center about two hours from where I lived, so I was already down with the theory—and even the practice—of meditation. After I had Maia, however, the idea of sitting down, undisturbed, for even five or ten minutes seemed ridiculous. Hell, it *was* ridiculous.

And yet the suggestion kept coming up.

First a good friend of mine started going to therapy. Her therapist's prescription? A book called *Wherever You Go, There You Are* by Jon Kabat-Zinn. My friend then headed over to the hospital to see if she could get her hands on some Prozac or Valium. The result? A referral to the "Meditation Specialist." The whole thing started getting closer to home when the same *Wherever You Go . . .* book on meditation mysteriously appeared in *my* apartment. Every self-help book I picked up, even the ones that didn't look too wind-chimey and scary, seemed to start with the suggestion that if I didn't meditate, everything else I could do for myself was futile. Pretty soon it seemed as if every somewhat stable person I came into contact with, if questioned long enough, would admit that she meditated with some kind of regularity. I found all of this totally unsettling (as did my friend, who could not get a Valium prescription for the life of her).

Maybe it's just me, but when I feel that something is going wrong in my life, I want to *do* something about it. At some point, however, I had to resign to my meditative fate. I'm not talking about sitting cross-legged for hours on end chanting "om," although you can do that too. I'm talking about just sort of being. And there are a million different ways to just sort of be. You can try a walking meditation where you don't go anywhere in particular. You can resolve to wake up a little earlier than your kids do and sit at the kitchen table letting your thoughts drift up and away without judging anything that goes through your mind. You can pick up one of Natalie Goldberg's writing books and take up "free writing" as your meditation. You can watch the sunset—just watch it. Even if your baby is up, you can try unplugging the phone for an hour and just relaxing to whatever's going on. The means you use to relax aren't important; just do whatever it takes to make you feel calm in the madness. As they say in *Shambala Warrior Training*, the first thing to "do" when you wake up and realize that you're having a nervous breakdown is to relax and be kind to yourself: It is, after all, a "basically good nervous breakdown."

"I've Been Unexpectedly Called Away"

Even though our mental crises can be even more important to deal with than our physical health or other family emergencies, telling our bosses, clients, or professors that we're having a nervous breakdown can be pretty taboo. Honesty, in these situations, is overrated. If you are dealing with people who aren't going to help you out—people whom you just have to cancel meetings with—feel free to lie.

"I've been unexpectedly called out of town on a family emergency" is a nice story. It's not really a lie either, considering that your sanity may very well be a "family emergency" and "out of town" can be either geographical or psychological. The cool thing about this one is that you can put it on your answering machine for all who would bother you, and no one is likely to ask about the details. They will think that some embarrassing thing has happened to your uncle, and they probably won't be terribly pushy about getting the whole story.

Another good story is that you are sick. This also isn't really a lie, but people will presume that you are talking physical breakdown. Be careful with this one, though. If you are having a manic episode and cavorting around town on some kind of high-heel-extreme-femme craze, folks might begin to wonder. But what the hell, they've probably wondered all along.

Also, if you answer the phone at all while you are "sick" and wanting people to believe that it's physical, make sure you sound stuffed-up, far away, and basically illin'.

Redesigning Your Life

Life as a mom is intrinsically crazy-making, but there are things we can do to avoid too many gnarly episodes. The aforementioned meditation is good. One of my neighbors, who has a large tribe of children, screams "I am not these responsibilities" in the shower every morning. Prayer works too. If you don't believe in any kind of higher power, try praying to your ancestors, or make some goddess-saint up. I myself am partial to the unofficial "Saint Erma Bombeck." The only requirement for being an object of reverence, in my opinion, is that the image cannot look anything like that evil middle school principal who punished you for telling your almost-as-evil social studies teacher where to go. We're talking about a compassionate higher power, all right?

The point of prayer is, essentially, to take the burden off you and make you feel happy, peaceful, and comforted, so even if you're not down with God, Erma, or the Virgin, doing something like redecorating a room with soothing colors or planting a garden might have a similar effect.

Cutting down on all the shit you have to do will also help enormously. I am not an expert on this, as I have to finish a draft of this book by next week, put out a magazine in three days, edit another newsletter over the weekend, cohost a radio show on Friday, plan a national week of resistance to stop the war on mothers and children, not to mention the fact that I'm supposed to be having some semblance of a family life. This, I solemnly warn you, is a recipe for disaster (and may explain why I have to pray so much). Since I've reached total overload, however, I'm starting to "just say no," and it's very cool. Make a list of all the "responsibilities" you can either delegate or get out of all together, and then go for it—clear your calendar. Start being reasonable about what you can do. If you still have too much to do, pick up a copy of *Simplify Your Life* by Elaine St. James for ideas or, at least, get in the habit of screaming "I am not these responsibilities" in the shower every morning.

In the meantime, be kind to yourself and take care of your physical health. Drink a lot of water. Don't eat Cheese Whiz. Exercise. Don't walk around muttering "I am a total dork." Get as much sleep as you can possibly get away with. Electricity is not a natural thing—we humans are supposed to be in bed from sunset to sunrise. Try to do the natural sleep thing at least once a week.

If you are still hanging out with any negative or energy-sucking people, diss them now. The test is "Do I feel worse after I spend time with this person than I did before?" If the answer is even a somewhat consistent "yes," inform them that you need to take a little break from the relationship—like fifty years.

Cut down on your work hours if at all possible. Working forty hours per week is not natural or fun. If you are working more than that, you are asking for trouble. If you're working too much just to pay the bills, please join me and my ragtag revolutionary army: We intend to overthrow the current capitalistic, patriarchal system that forces us mamas to work too hard and have too many nervous breakdowns. If you are working too much because you are a workaholic or you really think you need to be making $400-a-month car payments and going to the mall every time you get an hour off, get a grip. Repeat three times after me: "My sanity is worth more than this paycheck. My sanity is worth more than this car. My sanity is worth more than that cute velvet bra from Victoria's Secret. My sanity is worth more than this fucking job!"

Daily Affirmations for Crazed Moms

- I am not these responsibilities.

- I deserve to be happy and sane.

- I am an awesome mom.

- Everyone who thinks otherwise can just kiss my rosy red ass.

- I am a glorious daughter of Saint Erma Bombeck.

- I do not have to overthrow the government *this week*.

- No, I cannot make five dozen brownies for your fucking PTA meeting!

~~~~~~~~~~~~~~~~~

Rebel Mom

"Prozey," the Depression Doll

Tamar Spiegelman-Kern, mama of one

I know you were depressed for over a year—tell us about the beginning of that time.

Well, we were living in Germany when I got pregnant. I loved it there, but my husband got super sick. I wanted to stay in Germany, but because of his health we really had to go back to Ithaca, New York. I was doing everything by myself and I didn't even know if my husband was going to live to see his child. He was having all these tests done because they didn't know what was wrong with him.

Finally, some of their treatments started working and he started getting better, but then he got offered a job, and so he was gone all the time. Our families didn't know any of this was going on, so I felt very alone.

One night when my husband was feeling okay, we went out and we got in a big fight and I just cried and cried. I cried so hard I thought I was going to lose the baby. I got in the shower to try and stop crying, but I was just heaving and heaving. Those were the first symptoms—I cried so much sometimes, all I could feel was sadness. When I was being loved and supported by the people around me, I couldn't feel the support. I could only feel heartache.

I was in labor for three days, so my husband took all of his maternity leave to walk around Ithaca with me. Then Atticus was born on a Friday, and my husband had to go back to work on Monday.

So you were alone again.

Well, two days later all of our families arrived, about twenty visitors. So I had this five-day-old infant and I was making tea for people. They would say "go rest," but I couldn't. I would get into bed, but I would hear their voices and I couldn't sleep.

Was this classified as a postpartum depression?

No. I was depressed postpartum, but it had started when I was pregnant and continued for about a year after he was born. Postpartum depression is really that hormonal, chemical thing that happens after you have a baby. For me, that whole first year was really hard. It wasn't totally hormonal, although that didn't help. It also didn't help that Atticus didn't sleep through the night until he was nine months old. The weather in that part of the country didn't help either. There were two blizzards when Atticus was a baby.

In one way it was a really sweet time. Atticus was a baby and my friend who had lived in Thailand would come over every day and make Thai soup. But it was also a really hard time. I went down to a place where I had never been before. It was a dark time.

What did you do?

Well, when you have this little baby, you can't indulge yourself in moodiness and sadness. You really can't just stay in bed and watch *Oprah* or be cosmically depressed when you've got this little baby looking up at you. In a way, Atticus really gave me the strength and the motivation to deal with the depression head on, because I knew I had to be there for him. I kept it together as much as I could. I did therapy. I tried herbs. But I didn't want to do drugs because I was nursing. I went to this Jungian and she said, "You're on an ice floe and you can either start walking or stay still, but you are still going to be on this ice floe in the middle of the ocean." You know the Jungians, they just want you to sit with your sadness, but I was like, *Fuck you, I don't wanna feel like this.*

If someone came to you now in the same state you were in then, what would you tell them?

You just have to go through it. Things help. Reading about other women's experiences helps, especially if you can find someone to read about who is worse off than you. Then you can think, *Well, she's a nutcase, but I'm doing okay.*

I also went to an astrologist. That was cool. That sort of takes the responsibility off you and puts it on the universe. She said it was the Saturn Return because I was thirty, so I thought, *Okay, this is the Saturn Return. This is not because I am a weak, degenerate, soulless freak.*

Part of it for me was realizing how different I was now that I was a mom. I couldn't quite be that same giggly Patty Duke–like character. In a way that was good. It made it impossible for me to keep being a chameleon and keep presenting whatever side of Tamar was expected at a certain moment. I had to get real.

It would have been super awesome if I had had a friend who had a baby right at the same moment I did, but I didn't. Family is supposed to be helpful too, but, you know, my mom was forever putting one of those "pee pee stopper" pads down wherever I would sit with the baby and putting diapers down for burping. It was all a little too complicated for me.

My husband and Atticus were totally there for me, though. My husband never flinched, he was never like "Why don't you take an aerobics class? You'll feel better." So I realized I didn't have to be this *uber*-mom. I was just Tamar.

Did you ever end up taking Prozac?

Yes. I went to see this psychotherapist who charged me $450 for a forty-five-minute hour, and then he wanted to see me the next week for another $225. He wouldn't take any insurance. You can only get Prozac if you have the cash. I had to mortgage my life to get that drug. Then I went to fill the prescription and the pharmacist was looking at me with his pitiful dog eyes, like *Oh you poor psych ward child,* but I got the drug.

Have you ever floated in a salt lake? You can't sink. Even if you swim down deep, you float back up. That's what Prozac is like. I didn't cry when I was taking it, which was weird for me because I always cry. It also completely reversed the effect of PMS. But even with all those great things happening, I didn't like it. It takes a few notes off the top and a few notes off the bottom. You don't feel the low, but you don't feel the same happiness either. So I stopped taking it after a couple of months.

So how did you get back up without the drug?

When Atticus was about a year old it just started lifting. There was this woman who did a postpartum depression group in Rochester, New York, and she said that it would go away, but that I would never be quite the same. I was scared when she said that, but it has turned out to be true. It has changed me forever. I am more compassionate, and stronger. I'm so strong now, I can lift a car with my nose.

The bad part of that change is that now the road to that deep, black, bottom hole is very well marked. Now keeping that from happening again is important.

How do you keep it from happening?

I go to lots of movies. I think I have an overflow of emotions. You know, some people have an overflow of brains and they are too smart? I have an overflow of emotions so I just have to cry. I cry at every movie I see. I cry at the previews. And I eat a lot of chicken.

Chicken?

Yeah. I am convinced that they shoot chickens up with all these hormones that somehow bring me an inner calm. It's better than meditation or sex or anything. Chicken.

Tell me about Prozey, the depression doll you made.

Prozey just happened one day. I love my Prozey. She has cool hair, because that's my one claim to fame. Cool hair. She is full of beans. She's not stuffed quite right. She has dolphins in the back of her mind. Her heart is on her sleeve. And she has nice shoes. She has a cape of hooks. That was weird. Everybody loved Prozey until they saw her cape of hooks and then they were like, *This is weird.*

The hooks are about getting caught on people and things, caught on sadness, and being hypersensitive, but hooks can also catch you when you are falling. Inside the cape I made it really cool. There are angels, because underneath depression there is love. I sewed Prozac into the hem of the cloak. I think that was some kind of Nazi Germany trip, like *If things get really bad, I can just take my Prozey and flee!*

Tamar never did have to flee, and you probably won't either. Nervous breakdowns are usually temporary, but they signal a time for us to take better care of ourselves.

Chapter 10

Poverty Without Despair

"Um, ma'am, we haven't received a payment from you since 1994." —Working Assets operator on why my long distance service was cut off

"If worse comes to worst," says Holly, a thirty-two-year-old mother of four, "I just sit out on the street with a sign and read somebody's palm."

In the more than five years Holly and her kids have lived without any steady income, she's also been known to sell T-shirts on the street, borrow the money for a classified ad and throw a spontaneous tag sale, go through her photographs of her children and sell the best ones as postcards, and haggle with the landlord and phone and electric companies with a sweet voice and persuasive tone.

Like one in ten women who go through a divorce, Holly was left penniless and homeless after her marriage ended. She and her four preschoolers turned to friends and family for help but finally ended up in a shelter.

"I don't even know how I dealt with it," Holly admits now. "But I just refused to give up. I had to have a positive attitude. We were in this new place, so I just tried to make it fun for the kids. I said to myself, 'No matter what, I can't let anybody fuck my poor little kids' heads up.' And I waited until they were asleep to really try to deal with myself and get a grip."

While it isn't always true that poverty is less stressful for people who are used to being poor, it is true that poverty is less stressful for people who are resourceful, for people who don't have "too much pride" to talk to their landlord about the situation, and for people who refuse to despair, no matter what. And oh yeah—for people who know how to read palms.

Even if you haven't hit rock bottom, it can't hurt to be prepared: Some of the strategies learned in the trenches of poverty can be helpful to anyone, so read on.

Buying Time

The time to take action is *before* a major crisis hits. Once you've got an eviction notice or your electricity has been shut off, you will probably be dealing with some very annoyed and uncompassionate-seeming people who are holding all the cards. So see if you can't talk to the folks who are expecting a check in the mail from you.

The truth is always—well, usually—a good place to start. Explain your situation to your creditors, your landlord, and your utility company reps. Don't fall into the bottomless "I'm embarrassed and the situation is hopeless" pit—that can be a pretty hard one to climb out of. Sure, telling the truth might turn out to be a waste of time, but you never know when your hard-ass attorney-accountant landlord will start having flashbacks to his own homeless childhood and show a little compassion. Failing that, he probably has a pretty good idea of how

Some Cool Things About Poverty

- No worries about "spoiling" your kids.
- Historically, you are in excellent company. Try to think of ten great women in history who never lived in poverty.
- No one will ask to borrow money.
- Makes for good memoirs.
- No taxes.
- Nothing left to lose.
- Don't have to balance your checkbook anymore.
- Telemarketers will stop calling after a while.

hard it is to evict someone. (Call your local tenants' rights association to find out the rules that will apply to you, but if *my* landlord tried to evict me, it would take him three, long, rent-free months.)

The only approach I would absolutely discourage in dealing with creditors is calling the woman who telephones you about your over-due bills a "professional bitch." I'll spare you the details, but when I tried this one, the result was *very* ugly.

Utility companies, and even landlords, are often happy to set up some kind of payment plan with you. Obviously, if there isn't going to be any money coming in the foreseeable future, this doesn't sound so great, but buy as much time as you can. Try not to get all worried and kiss-butt on the phone and tell them you'll have it by the end of the week if you really don't think you will. But if this is the best deal you can cut, it's better than no time at all. In bill- and rent-paying negoti-

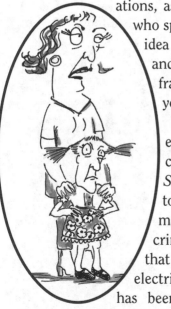

ations, as in other negotiations, remember that she who speaks first loses. In other words, try to get an idea of how hard-ass your creditor is going to be, and try to get *them* to suggest a payment time frame before you go and offer some deal that you're not going to be able to pull off.

If you discover that the truth just isn't good enough for whoever you're dealing with, you can try following Sarah Dunn's advice. In *The Slacker Handbook* she suggests bullshitting to the tune of claiming you have a dead house-mate, claiming that your place is a bona fide crime scene, convincing the utility companies that you have some dread disease you need the electricity on for, or telling them that your place has been quarantined by your local Health and Human Services department.

Fictional checks tend to slow the process down a little too. This should be a last resort, however, as the bank will take the opportunity to charge you another small fortune for bouncing the check, and once your creditor gets a bad check from you, you are in a much worse legal situation. But, hey, the lights will be on until everyone catches on.

I am presuming here, of course, that you are not even worrying about consumer debt, student loans, and the like. But you can tell those folks the truth too. Try something like "And bad credit has caused *how many* fatalities in the past year?"

Confessions of a Collection Agent

I recently convinced a collection agent I know that perhaps she could clear her conscience by sharing a few insights into the trade with all of us Hip Mamas. So what did she have to say?

Well, "You are supposed to be able to tell a collection agent to stop calling you and, legally, they have to stop, but do you think we record those conversations? No. Tell the collection agent you are going to pay so they will give you their address, then send them a letter and tell them to stop calling you. You can also 'CC' the attorney general, then we will definitely stop harassing you."

And then what will you do to us?

"Not a lot," she says. "We can sue. We can attach your assets. We can take your car, but we hardly ever do because we figure you don't own it anyway. We can attach your bank account if we know where it is, but if you don't really have anything, well, there are no debtor's prisons."

But what happens if you sue us?

"Not a lot," she admits again. "The student loan collectors have more resources and more rights than consumer or business collection agents, and if you've written a bad check we can sue you for treble damages so your $50 check will now be a $5,000 court-ordered payment, but what are we going to do with a court order if you have no money? You've already told us to stop calling you. All we can do is ruin your credit for seven years. Big deal."

Hmm . . . any other advice?

"Yes, pay your necessities, then your car, then your student loans, and then worry about anything else. If you own a business, incorporate. We screw the sole proprietors and the partners, but if you are incorporated you just close the business and open another, and we can't touch you. I'm good at my job because I can be very aggressive and make people think I'm holding all the cards, but in reality, it's a rare case when I can do a damn thing about anybody's debts. Also, I work on commission. I'll give up if it is clear to me that you are not going to pay."

Ten Quick Ways to Come Up with $10 to $100 Without Selling Your Body

The following quick fixes will seem obvious to the experienced poor person, but some of them took me a while to figure out, so I thought I'd pass 'em on to those of you who are new to the trenches.

1. Have a garage sale. Advertise in the paper only if you have enough stuff so you know you'll recover the expenses. Otherwise, bright signs around town will do.

2. Go around your neighborhood asking everyone for their old shit, then take it to the flea market. Get there early enough to sell a lot of the stuff off to other vendors. Professional flea-marketers won't pay you as much for things, but they are willing to sit there with the crap for weeks on end waiting for it to sell. If you don't have money for a stall, just get there really early and sell to other vendors. (Find your local site under "Flea markets" or "Swap meets" in the Yellow Pages.)

3. Call the Salvation Army, the United Way, local churches, and every other agency listed in your phone book under "Community Services," "Emergency Services," and "Women's Organizations" and tell them what's up.

4. Call your grandmother.

5. Eat out and then tell them the food was so disgusting, there's no way you're paying for it. Bringing dead flies and/or hair to throw on the food you don't eat can help.

6. Offer to wash people's car windows in a bustling parking lot. This takes some serious hustling skills, but with enough fast talking, it may bring in up to $20 an hour.

7. Get familiar with the resale value of books and children's clothes at your local resale shop; buy stuff at garage sales that you are relatively certain will go for more downtown.

8. Get a small garage band together. If you're good, pass a hat. If you suck, put up a sign that says you will stop playing for five minutes for every dollar you get.

9. If you haven't already, apply for welfare. Don't forget to ask about any emergency money you may be eligible for.

10. If you own anything from J. Crew, Tweeds, Nordstrom, or any other store with an unconditional return policy, return it! Unconditional means just what it says. I once returned an ugly and shrunken five-year-old sweater to Tweeds. My grandmother will break out in a cold sweat when she reads this, but Tweeds ain't gonna miss the $40.

The Art of Denial

As Mary Kay Blakely has pointed out, "Young children's capacity for denial is enormous." When her family's electricity and phone got cut off, she just acted as if everyone lived in the dark sometimes. And actually, most people do at one time or another. It's not all that cool to lie, but kids get pretty sick of the old "We don't have any money" sob story. Any other vaguely sincere explanation will do. It has only very recently occurred to me, for example, that when my mom helped us decorate a lemon tree in the front yard the Christmas I was four, her story about "this is how they did it in the olden days" was a total afterthought. In reality, Christmas trees were incredibly expensive, and we'd already cut down and made off with the local country club's tree the year before. This isn't the kind of bullshit kids usually grow up to resent.

I realize that the concept of denial has lost some of its popularity in recent years, but we don't *always* have to deal in reality. Doesn't "vegetarians are healthier" sound better than "we can't afford any meat"?

Beth, a twenty-nine-year-old welfare mom, tells her kids that food stamps are a kind of lottery winning. Another mom I know acts as if picking up all the free furniture she sees on the street is simply a more convenient way to shop—like getting your burgers at the drive-through instead of going inside.

I've noticed that this cheerful reflex comes easier to some of us. A lot of moms who are new to the whole poverty thing feel the need to comment on their own lack of cash whenever they think of it. But we could all learn something from our kids' enormous capacity for denial. I mean, eating vegetarian *is* healthier, food stamps *are* a kind of prize, and picking up whatever crap is on the street is a hell of a lot more convenient than going to Sears—forget your primary motivations. I had a blast decorating that lemon tree when I was four, and if my mom's got a regret list anywhere, I hope that Christmas tree isn't on it.

I recently made a list of my bare essential expenses (rent, utilities, food, and transportation plus $20 a week) and I couldn't help laughing when I realized I had lived on about 60 percent of the total for the first six years of Maia's life. I am not at all certain how I did this, but one trick I learned early on was *not* to write these things down. Budgeting is for people who have at least some remote hope of being able to afford their bare essentials. The rest of us just have to figure out how to pay the rent. Running water, gas, and electricity are nice too. But it won't kill you to be without a phone for a while—and having your phone disconnected usually cuts down on collection-agent harassment. Think: *Little House on the Prairie*, and be *really* careful if you're using candles or trying to cook on some camp stove contraption. In fact, just sleep when it gets dark and go for cold food. Propane is scary.

What Poor People Know

- Their landlord/lady's disposition. Talk to them, talk to them, talk to them. No landlord wants to have to evict you.
- Their tenants' rights.
- Their utility companies' cut-off policies.
- Fictional checks, while sometimes necessary, are how banks make an amazing amount of money off poor people.

- Check cashing places are even worse than banks. Get a little savings account at a real bank where you can cash checks.
- If you need emergency shelter or food, go to the mayor's office. Mayors hate having homeless people in their hallways and can often get you a bed in a supposedly "full" shelter.
- If you put a one-cent stamp on a letter or bill and leave off your return address, the receiver will be charged the postage. (If you put no postage on the envelope, it will not be delivered.)
- Many long-distance companies are so desperate for customers that they will hook you up even if you owe one of their competitors money. (But be careful with AT&T or other long-distance companies that bill through your local company.)

Finding Outside Resources

All right, we need to get you some cash, girlfriend. We're on a mission. Start by doing something soothing—take some deep breaths, take a hot bath if you've still got water, and see if you can, at least for the day, take a sort of Zen approach to your life. A lot of folks will judge you when you don't have any money—please don't join them. It is the economy, not your character, that is fundamentally flawed. I don't care how you got into this situation; in a decent society, it would be *impossible*.

Anyway, back to our mission. I'm going to start pretty high on the food chain, here, so if the first few ideas make you laugh hysterically, just bear with me. Get out a pen and paper. Where can you get money, food, or other assistance? Begin with any personal resources you can cash in. Do you have any savings? Spending it is a much better personal-finance move than maxing out your credit cards. Do you own a car worth more than $2,000? If so, sell it and buy a cheaper one. Are you making car payments? No matter what your financial situation, car payments are a big ripoff—so give the cute new eggplant-color minivan back and pick up something with a little more, uh, *character*. Do you own anything else you can sell? Obviously you don't want to shoot yourself in the foot here. I mean, if you're a writer, selling your computer is an extremely bad move, but if you're a musician, then selling your camera equipment might not be so terrible.

Do you have any weird savings or stock accounts that your great-grandmother told you not to cash in until 2050? Cash 'em in!

Do you have an extraordinary amount of debt? You might want to consider filing for bankruptcy. It will ruin your credit, but contrary to popular belief, many of us live perfectly normal lives with really shitty credit.

Once you've assessed your own situation and done as much as you feel you can do to get yourself out of the throes of poverty, make a list of any family members or friends who are likely to help you out without too many strings attached. If you are going to call funds from people you know "loans," please be honest with them about their chances of getting repaid within the next five years.

Call your local Social Services and find out what the current status of welfare is. Ask about food stamps and health insurance too.

Next, go through your phone book and write down all the numbers for community services, women's services, and religious organizations in your area. Call them. Call the mayor's office. Many agencies do not give cash directly to poor people (because they think we'll spend it on beer and crack . . . *as if!*), so be clear about what you need—is it shelter, food, clothing, child care, utility payments, rent money, legal aid, Christmas toys, or all of the above? Write down what each agency can offer you. Expect a certain amount of buck-passing and dead-end referrals, but remember that asking a church if it has a free-food program is no weirder than calling a school and asking if it has financial aid, or calling Tower Records and asking if they have the new Bikini Kill CD. If you are not treated with respect, keep your head held high and complain. Thank people who are nice to you, but remember that you would do the same for them.

Once you've got a few checks coming from relatives and have made contact with, shall we say, your major potential funders, it's time to visit them.

The welfare office will probably be your first stop. The wait may be long, the bureaucracy unnerving, and the ambiance in the waiting room seriously lacking, but welfare is still your best bet. You will probably have to fill out separate applications for food stamps, medical coverage, and cash aid, and all of these things will take a long time, but they may be well worth it. Remember when you are filling out the application that you have to be honest, but you don't have to be *painfully* honest. A good rule of thumb is that you have nothing and you know no one. When I filled out my first application for food stamps, they asked if I prepared meals communally with anyone. Thinking that would be a good idea, I almost marked "yes." Luckily, an experienced food stamp mama sitting across from me warned that I would not be eligible for any food stamps, no matter how poor I was, if I marked the dreaded "yes" box. "You have nothing, and you know no one," she advised.

If you have questions about welfare or other resources that may, depending on the answer, be incriminating, ask them on the phone and do not give your name.

Next, you'll want to go around to the churches and other organizations that you've contacted. In my experience, church people tend to be very kind, but I do try to avoid sharing too many of my political opinions with folks who are feeding me. It is likely that a church worker will tell you something like "God bless you," which I'm sure you can deal with, but you should never be made to feel that you have to convert to some weird born-again thing in order to eat.

Finally, even if you've gotten an iffy response on the phone from the mayor's office, please head over to city hall. Once elected officials have homeless families in their offices (especially those who calmly mention how interested the local newspaper will be in the issue), they will come up with *something*.

Child Support

If you are a single mom and there's someone out there with potential or established paternity rights, you are entitled to get some child support. Unless you are dealing with a batterer or someone who is so low-income that it couldn't possibly do you any good to get a court order, there aren't very many good reasons to forgo suing for support. If you apply for welfare, the county may be in charge of collecting your support. This can be a very slow process, but you can help speed things up by sending regular updates about your child's father's whereabouts and helping them out in any other way you can.

Whatever your situation, learn about child support laws and enforcement of those laws by requesting a five-dollar information kit from the NOW Legal Defense and Education Fund at (212) 925-6635 and a free Child Support Enforcement Information Package from the folks at Child Support Enforcement at (202) 401-9383. You can also call your state child support enforcement office, which should be listed in the government pages of your phone book.

Child support orders are generally based on a complicated formula that takes into account your income, your child's father's income, how many children each of you has to support, and, in some states, the amount of time your children spend with each of you. This can add up to a pretty big chunk of money. So find out how much money you are looking at and fight for it.

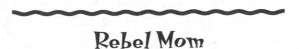

Rebel Mom

Shamama's in the House

Shamama Motheright (a.k.a. Siobhan Lowe-Matuk),
poverty consultant and visionary mama of four

So, what is a poverty consultant?

I call myself a consultant in American poverty. We are all consultants in poverty. Some people go to college, some people experience a different lifestyle called "survival," and in that process we come up with inspirations and solutions that will relieve our country's tired economic system.

Can you describe your education in survival to me?

The isolation as a mother brought about in me an absolute fervor to get to know others like me. I knew I could not be the only one of my kind. I was living in total Appalachian backwoods, in Tennessee, in

West Virginia, and in Sharon, Pennsylvania, five blocks from a steel mill and two blocks from the toughest crack ghetto in the state. It was there among a lot of the fifteen-year-old mommies that I started to run my mouth off my front porch.

Instead of "not in my backyard," it was "naturally in my backyard." So I got these girls to plant gardens all through the neighborhood. They knew me as "Sister Tie-dye" back then.

Then, magically, I was transported to Floyd, Virginia, where there is an eclectic group of evolutionist women—I don't say revolutionist, because that's a little too butch for me. In Floyd I was doing things like chopping wood to stay warm and dealing with water from old funky pipes. Being so far out rurally allowed for a speeded-up consciousness. Even though I got a check that was only $300 a month for four kids, I could make my own rules rurally.

And you began to evolve into the visionary Shamama . . .

Well, sister-girlfriend, this is the vision in full psychedelic Technicolor: combine welfare checks; combine Section Eight housing grants; find land—there is tons of it; and, in trust, build these houses out of old tires, beer cans, and straw bales. It sounds crazy, but check out Dennis Weaver. He's a rich movie star who lives in one of these houses. It's totally buff. It's totally solar. It's warm and dry, and these are good things that we women go without.

We will need to get some muscle to help build these houses, so we get the people who are in jail owing money for child support to be let out and to come work off their debt by building these homes alongside the women who want to live in them.

These would be communities built on healing and shared labor. And they would be a gift to give back to the American taxpayers who took care of us when no one else would.

Imagine on-site child care, good food grown in the gardens. We could also invite politically correct, environmentally friendly corporations to build nearby—like Ben and Jerry's—I'd say, *yeah, c'mon down here, babies.* There is no limit to how this could relieve our country, and there is no limit to the joy and self-pride with which we would give this gift back to America—the country we live in, the country we love. We are not patriots, though. We are matriots. It's a mother's right to dream a new future into reality.

Sounds very cool. What's the current status of all of this?

It's beginning to catch on here and there. The more people hear about it, the more people place ads in the newspaper for poor mothers to come and meet. It's hard because a lot of people feel like "It's too much, I can't do that," but I feel in my heart that we as mothers can pull this off—in a historical way, like new pioneers.

Word on the street is that you've also started a new political party.

Yes. Motheright. I say, *Hey, y'all Washington, D.C., Republicans and you necktie-too-tight Democrats. You need to slide over, boys, 'cause the Motherights are in the house.* It's a Mother's right to believe she can create change for all the mothers out there.

Do you have any advice for mamas who are new to poverty?

Yes. Take the newfound poverty as the ultimate challenge—as the coolest game you've ever played to get back at the system. Whittle away at yourself and your need for fu-fu items. Find the yard sales and the garage sales. They are glory lands. Church sales are cool too. You can get real quality clothing—to hell with K-Mart. Check out food in bulk, and store food. If you can have a garden, that's the best because you can can-up. I canned up three hundred jars of food from the garden this summer and I've been eating all winter. It's medicine food because it has the vibes from the summer. Another thing I've been doing is cutting up Juicy Juice cans and making beautiful goddess mobiles that people want to buy. We can make art out of garbage.

Ask yourself what you really need and challenge yourself to go without and still be centered and secure minimalistically. And whatever you do, don't demean yourself. You wouldn't let a bunch of funky drunk crackheads into your living room, so neither should you give self-deprecatory, negative, ca-ca thoughts free rent in your head—

no, no, no—you're part of an exciting explosion of showing the American people that you can make it and fight in spite of it all.

As long as we don't give all those self-deprecating thoughts free rent in our minds, poverty can be a radicalizing instead of debilitating experience. So keep on keeping on . . .

Chapter 11

Surviving Family Breakup

"A good divorce is better for children than a bad marriage.   —Ashton Applewhite,* Cutting Lose

Samantha knew her relationship with her baby's father was over. She saw the signs, cried after the screaming arguments, felt the dull pain and disappointment and dread that come before the inevitable end. Still, she tried to ignore it all. She was finishing her senior year in college, busy with the new baby, tired all the time. She figured they'd straighten things out later.

"Then I came home from school one day and they were gone," she remembers. "He had asked me to fill the gas tank up and cash his paycheck the day before, but I didn't think anything of it. All of a sudden I was standing there in the entryway, leaking milk, ready to nurse the baby, thinking *They're gone*. I just stood there for I don't know how long, and finally a process server showed up and handed me a custody suit."

For most of us, the end of a relationship is less dramatic than what happened to Samantha, but every divorced mother remembers the moment of shock when she realized it was really over.

Emergency Action

If you are being sued for divorce or child custody, if you or your children are the victims of domestic violence, or if you need an emergency court order for child custody or visitation, take a deep breath. You can handle this. But you don't have time to process the whole experience just yet. Family law emergencies are like blazing house fires—you have to remain calm, stay low to the floor, get your family out of the building, and grieve your losses later.

If you or your children are in immediate danger, take all the money you have, all legal papers—IDs, birth certificates, social security cards, and so on—and whatever else you have time to grab (like the children's security toys or blankets) and run. If you don't have a friend's house or shelter to go to, the police station or, worst-case scenario, an all-night restaurant will do. Keep calm, frame the situation as an adventure for the kids, forget what you saw on the "Movie of the Week," and remember that you survived labor—and you will survive this.

Once you're working from a place of safety, the first step, according to California family law attorney Linda French, is to assess the situation with an expert. You can find an expert by looking under "Attorneys, Family Law," "Women's Organizations," or "Community Services" in the Yellow Pages. Your local "Commission on the Status of Women" or YWCA are also good places to call for referrals, or check the "Survival Notes" in the back of this book for national hot-line numbers. As you are calling around, make sure to ask about free or low-cost legal services in your community if you think you'll need them.

What you probably need is a family law attorney or a paralegal counselor who is used to dealing with family law. (A tax lawyer is useless in a custody case.) If a crime has been committed, you need to file a police report immediately.

If you have a real emergency, you will need to get some temporary court orders for custody and/or protection. An attorney or the staff at a women's shelter can help you get the orders you need, and the police and the district attorney's office can help you enforce the orders.

If you have been served with divorce or custody papers, you can represent yourself in court, but you probably should get a sense of your legal standing by seeing an attorney. Generally you will have a couple of weeks to prepare for your hearing, but the court can issue emergency orders within about twenty-four hours.

If your child or children have been kidnapped by their other parent, you will need as much legal backup as you can possibly afford. Unless there is an existing court order, either parent may be able to take the children away for as long as he or she wishes. You will likely need an emergency custody order establishing your parental rights before the police will help you find the kids.

A retainer for full legal representation can cost up to about $2,500, but legal consultations are often free or available for $50 to $100.

Call friends and family to let them know what is going on. You might be surprised to find that they have either been through a similar ordeal or know of a valuable resource in your community. The same emergency has happened before. You are not alone.

Dealing with an unexpected divorce or custody emergency is like running a marathon without any training. Be good to yourself. Driving yourself crazy won't help the situation. Eat healthy foods when you're hungry, sleep when you're tired, and take a hot bath whenever you can. Miracles come after a lot of hard work, so remind yourself that you deserve one.

Some Cool Things About Family Breakup

- The loser is gone!

- Historically, you are in excellent company. Most great feminists have had great divorces.

- No one will think you're normal and square.

- Makes for good memoirs.

- Child support checks are fun to get.

- You will feel like a teenager as your name gets back in the gossip mill when your kid tells her teachers things like "My mommy did sexes with Bobby's dad!"

- Builds character.

- One less mouth to feed.

Avoiding Evil Judges and Hard-Ass Attorneys

In my opinion, virtually every family breakup scenario is best settled out of court. You might, through no fault of your own, end up sitting in a seriously uncomfortable chair that reminds you of some seedy movie house listening to a white-haired, Republican-voting judge who hates you dictate your family's fate. But this should never be Plan A.

Plan A should be to pick up a copy of Karen Winner's book, *Divorced from Justice*, and educate yourself about the very real bias against women that exists in family court. Then get on-line (at your local library if not in your study), and go to http://www.divorce-help.com, http://www.divorce-online.com, and http://www.nolo.com. These are awesome resources because they offer up-to-date and localized information and support for dealing with every facet of your divorce. At some point, you are going to want to consult with an attorney. But if you and your ex can work this thing out with only a couple of "third" parties, you're miles ahead of the rest of us, and you'll be a lot happier in the end.

But always remember: You have the right to have your case heard by a judge. Don't let anyone tell you otherwise.

If you're heading into what feels like a relatively friendly divorce, you'll want to pat yourself on the back and do your damnedest to keep it that way. If things are starting to get ugly, however, prepare for all hell to break loose, but know that there's still hope. No matter what your situation, you have, essentially, three things to lose. They are

- your money
- your kids
- your sanity

You should give sanity priority because neither custody of your children nor all the money in the world will do you any good if you are in restraints at the state hospital in line for some god-awful new-fangled "treatment." But let's start with the easy stuff.

Your Money

When it comes to divorce, the less money you have, the better. By your money, I mean all the cash, bank accounts, stocks, bonds, clothes, property, assets, businesses, books, land, cats, jewelry, big old papier-mâché statues of the Virgin Mary, homes, furniture, boats, trinkets, motorcycles, patents, old vinyl records, debts, future pensions, photographs, and every other nonhuman thing you or your ex have any claim to. Some of these things are easy to split up. The crap you moved in with is all probably still yours. And your ex's ratty old pile of shit you threw out the door and threatened to set fire to last month is probably still his. You don't need to document every old book that's in the house, but depending on how long you and your ex were together and how enmeshed your lives became, there's probably a pretty long list of "communal" items that fall somewhere in the expansive gray area. In theory, this vast collection of stuff that made up your coupled life is going to have to be split in an "equal," or at least "equitable," fashion. If you and your ex can agree on how to divide the money and the stuff, you don't have to follow any laws or guidelines. There are, however, a couple of standard ways divorcing couples usually split things up. The basic "equal distribution of assets" theory requires you to determine the fair market value of everything you've got, and either sell it all and split the proceeds or divide it so you each end up with a fair pile. You can begin to think about all of this by making three lists—your stuff, your ex's stuff, and that whole gray area.

If you've amassed a fair amount of property over the years, your list might look something like this:

Mine	His	Communal
Motorcycle	Stereo	House
Goofy art collection	Stamp collection	Stocks
Music collection (part)	Music collection (part)	VW
Cat	Rat	Computer
Powerbook	Boat	Furniture

As you read down the "communal" list, the first two things you'll probably notice are that (a) you have more than you thought you had, and (b) you want to keep it all. Let's say you think the kids shouldn't have to move, and (although we haven't gotten to the whole custody issue) you're planning to keep them, so you want the house. The furniture, you figure, also stays with the house. You need something more than your motorcycle to take them to school and back, so obviously you need the VW. You need to be able to work at home now, so you need the computer too. This is all good and fine if your ex is agreeable, you have massive amounts of money to pay him off, you agree to a low child support figure in exchange, and/or the stocks are worth an awful lot.

The long and short of all this is that it's going to get complicated. And you're going to want to play Liz Phair's "Exile in Guyville" over and over again until you can't stand her.

Studies show that despite "equitable distribution" and "community property" laws, women's standards of living go down by an average of 30 percent after a divorce and men's go up by an average of 10 to 15 percent. If you can beat those odds with a settlement, you'll probably want to go ahead with it.

If you can't come up with an agreement that both you and your ex can live with (few can), you'll want to get some help from one or more of these folks:

- **An appraiser:** She can straighten out disagreements about what everything's worth. Find her in the Yellow Pages or by calling the American Society of Appraisers at (800) 272-8258 or the Appraisal Institute at (312) 335-4100.

- **A financial planner:** She can help you figure out weird things like the value of future pensions and the tax consequences of various financial maneuvers. Find her in the Yellow Pages.

- **A financial mediator:** The mediator may or may not be the same person you'll want to go to for help figuring out how you are going to share custody of your kids, but either way, you can get a referral for a mediator by calling the Society of Professionals in

Dispute Resolution at (202) 783-7277 or the Academy of Family Mediators at (617) 674-2663.

The subject of financial as well as child-custody mediation will come up a lot as you're divorcing, so I should warn you about the problems with the system. Mediation, or the use of a neutral third party to help you and your ex negotiate an agreement, can indeed save you time, money, and abuse from the court system. The problem, however, is that mediation is done in private—there are no lawyers, no judges, no court reporters, and no chance for appellate review. Studies have shown that women are more likely than men to "give up" and agree to settlements they are not comfortable with in mediation. And in some states, mediation is a totally unregulated field without any standards at all. So be careful, and know your rights as a mother and a litigant before you go anywhere near a mediator's office.

Having said all of that, mediation can be an excellent choice if both parents are cooperative and just need a little help working through their anger to an agreement.

Your Kids

This is where things get difficult. There are no appraisers who can come in and tell you what your beautiful children are worth. It's considered pretty much universally bogus to split up the kids. And except with the rare very-young, very-easygoing child, a fifty-fifty custody split can be bad news for a little one's psyche. To make matters all the more heartbreakingly human, unless your children are unborn or very young, or unless your ex has committed some heinous crime or ditched the scene entirely, your kids have two parents, and they need to have a relationship with both of you. Before I lead you into a pit of despair, however, I should remind you that millions of us do manage to share custody without fucking our kids up. You can do it too.

I am presuming here that you are moving toward some kind of joint custody plan, but as I have mentioned before, men win 70 percent of litigated custody trials. Many women who go through horrible divorces end up thinking theirs were isolated incidents, even flukes. They are not. If your ex is seeking full custody and you don't want him to have it, be prepared to fight like hell.

Basically, when we talk about child custody, we're talking about legal custody as well as physical custody. Legal custody refers to who makes the religious, medical, educational, and other decisions about the children's upbringing. Physical custody refers to where and with whom the kids will live. In theory, whoever was the children's primary caregiver when the parents lived together should keep primary custody of them after the couple breaks up. Depending on what you and your ex want, the laws in your state, your relationship with your ex, and how far apart the two of you live, you have several options. You can have joint legal and joint physical custody, joint legal and sole physical custody, joint physical and sole legal custody, or whatever. When one parent has sole physical custody, the noncustodial parent usually gets some kind of visitation. This can range from one supervised afternoon a week (this is reserved for noncustodial parents of the heinous crime variety) to fully half of the days in the year. Here are ten pretty standard ways people I've talked to share custody of their children.

The "Reasonable Visitation" Plan:
When Robin and Mike divorced, he got full custody of the kids and Robin was granted "reasonable visitation," which meant she had the kids every weekend. Both parents, however, remained active in their daughters' school and other aspects of their daughters' lives, sharing joint legal custody.

The Hostility Plan:
Jonas and Beth harbor enough hostility toward each other that it would be detrimental to their daughter to have them talking on any regular basis. They live nearby, however, so visitation can be frequent. Their seven-year-old spends every other weekend (from Friday night through Monday morning) as well as every Wednesday afternoon with her father. Beth has sole legal and physical custody, but Jonas has access to their daughter's school and medical records, essentially so he can make sure Beth's not doing anything wildly different from what he would.

The Completely Out-of-Court Plan:
Maria and Veronica have one child, who is Lisa's biological offspring. The former couple has a good relationship and lived with

their son as coparents for the first four years of his life. Lisa has sole custody of him (they never went to court and Veronica has no legal claim to the child), but Lisa allows Veronica "reasonable visitation," which usually amounts to one or two weekends a month, a week in the summer, and evenings whenever it's convenient for both parents.

The Bicoastal Plan:

Judy and Bob live 3,000 miles apart, so Judy retains sole physical custody of their two children and Bob sees them for six weeks during the summer and one week over Christmas. Judy and Bob have a somewhat difficult relationship, but they are able to talk every few weeks when the children are out (sparing them the raised voices) and generally agree on upbringing issues, so they share joint legal custody. In addition to visiting their dad twice a year, the kids call him whenever they like. The couple has also agreed that when the kids hit their early teens, they will have the option of living school years with dad. (The teen years, I should note here, are likely to be so bizarre that there's really no use in worrying about them until they are upon you.)

The Flexible Plan:

Lecia and Terrance split up when their daughter was three, and the parents agreed to a fifty-fifty, joint legal and physical custody arrangement. Because Lecia's life has been in flux, however, and she has moved in and out of town several times, their now eight-year-old girl has spent some years living mostly with dad and some dividing her time more equally between her parents' homes. Lecia and Terrance readjust their arrangement as often as they need to and tend not to demand much of each other beyond understanding and general goodwill.

The Fifty-Fifty Plan:

Anna and Tom shared caring for their twin daughters with a kind of obsessive equality when they were married, so when the couple divorced they simply stayed living close by and split both legal and physical custody—shuttling the children back and forth between their homes every week. Since this proved to be an extremely hard gig, the whole gang got themselves into an ongoing support and mediation group where they could get regular professional help dealing with communication and keeping tabs on how their kids were holding up.

The "Dad's Back" Plan:
Mary Anne was never married to her son's father, and he showed little interest in the child for the first few years. When he came back asking for "reasonable visitation," the two finally agreed to visitation on a one-day-a-week fixed schedule.

The Stepparent Plan:
As a stepdad, Ron was a major part of his two stepsons' lives for only about two and a half years. The boys, ages four and eight, had grown very attached to him. When Ron moved out, he and Andrea, the boys' mother, agreed that he should have visitation once a week. This tapered off after several years, but it was a nice transition for the boys.

The Heinous Crime Plan:
Beverly and Jim divorced because Jim was violent both toward Beverly and toward their young son. After a lot of wrangling in court, the judge ordered that Jim's visits with the boy be supervised by his mother, and Beverly retained sole physical custody. The court split legal custody between the parents, so Jim retained a say-so in all decisions about their son's upbringing. Although Jim showed up for visits only sporadically and eventually contact tapered off, Jim's legal relationship with his son was never severed.

The Bird's Nest Plan:
For three years after they split up, Jennifer and Tony's three children remained in the family home, and their parents took turns moving in and out. This went on until everyone involved thought they would lose their marbles, after which they resorted to something similar to the "reasonable visitation" model.

Now, your eventual setup may or may not look anything like these "plans," but I should tell you that even the agreements that sound somewhat smooth took a lot of soul-searching, adjustments, surrendering, and tears to get to. They say that the average divorce storm of hostility, resentment, and general hell lasts five years, after which things get manageable. I know that five years sounds like a dreadfully long time, but I know very few families that have actually beat the odds. On the other hand, I don't know very many folks who have drawn it out much longer. My ex and I pretty much hold the record in terms of long-term hostility among the parents I've talked to, and even we have gotten to nods of acknowledgment rather than all-out war when we have the misfortune of running into each other unexpectedly.

Anyway, to decide on one of these plans while avoiding evil judges and hard-ass attorneys, you need to come to an agreement. "If we could agree on anything as major as child custody, we'd still be married," you're thinking. This is where the mediators come in. I need to draw a distinction again here between voluntary and mandatory mediation. Mandatory mediation exists in states like California and is often a crock of shit that's even worse than actually going to court. (If you can't come to an agreement, for example, the mediator decides for you, thus completely and totally blowing the whole point of mediation.) The mediation I'm talking about is where you and your ex sit down voluntarily and hammer out an agreement, and neither of you feels undue pressure to agree to things you are not comfortable with. Often mediators are also family law attorneys, but if they are not, they should recommend that each parent consult with an attorney before signing away any rights. In any case, supporters of this kind of mediation claim that it works in about 80 percent of cases—and in custody disputes, you can't do much better than that.

Before we leave the subject of mediation, I should also warn you not to bother if there's a history of domestic violence or if your relationship has been one in which you always end up giving in and going away feeling screwed. Studies show that women are much more likely to "give in" during mediation, and if, like many others I know, you know you'll fall into doormat behavior—be careful. It's a rare mediator who can help you negotiate your way out of a deep oppression. In cases like these you will probably *need* a hard-ass attorney to make up for your own soft ass.

Your Sanity

Last but not least, eh? Anything but least. The deal with your sanity is that it's both the easiest thing to lose track of and the only thing you can't do jack shit without. I should probably include your physical health in this category—as physical breakdowns tend to come sneaking up on you right in the middle of mental ones—but that goes without saying, no? As holistic and friendly as your divorce may be, family breakup is always a messy, depressing, stressful kind of hell. I've seen the toughest of gals buckle under. And as horrible as your relationship with your ex may have been, we all

Things to Remember in Mediation

- Although family mediators often look like therapists or good confidantes, they are not! Attempt not to be a basket case.
- Be businesslike and to the point.
- Stand up for what you think is best for your kids.
- If you can't talk to your ex without cussing, name-calling, and/or threats, address all of your comments to the mediator.
- If you have to go into mediation with a former batterer, demand separate meetings.
- If you agree to something, but then change your mind, *speak up!*
- Do not volunteer information that can be used against you later.

need time to grieve both the good moments and the lousy ones. In the midst of divorces, I've seen cantaloupes splattered all over living rooms, formerly easygoing folks chasing each other around with knives, sobbing breakdowns that lasted weeks, and pent-up anger get dumped on already-scared toddlers. I even know one chick who worked herself into a nine-day coma. Seriously. Many of us get so focused on the legal mess or emergency and on keeping our children comfortable that we forget to leave ourselves safe time to get angry, to grieve, and to reassess our lives.

If you don't already have a tough-as-hell support system in place when your family starts to split itself open and painfully transform right before your eyes, it's time to set one up. It doesn't have to be anything permanent or ideal right away. Just gather *all* of your resources. Call relatives (the ones who don't stress you out), friends, therapists, counselors, and confidential parental stress hot lines. Call baby-sitters, massage therapists, and that old roommate who was always so good at listening. Get into aromatherapy, take-out health food, long baths, meditation, yoga, or kickboxing. If you don't already have a therapist, start asking around for referrals. Check community bulletin boards, local newspapers, and the Internet for support groups.

You are going to make it through this, but you need to mother *yourself* as well as your children.

Music to Divorce By

Breakups and divorce, as I'm sure you've noticed, are so much fun that they are just about the only topic anyone ever sings about. If you find yourself short on truly rockin' divorce tunes, however, try these babes. You just might relate to them:

- Bikini Kill, *Reject All American*
- Ani DiFranco, *Dilate*
- Nina Hagen, *NunSexMonkRock*
- Hole, *Live Through This*
- Janis Joplin, *Greatest Hits*
- Alanis Morissette, *Jagged Little Pill*
- Liz Phair, *Exile in Guyville*
- Michelle Shocked, *Short, Sharp, Shocked*
- *Tank Girl* soundtrack
- Tina Turner, *What's Love Got to Do With It?*

Adventures in
Family Court

I know a heartbreaking number of women who have gotten royally screwed in family court, and often it doesn't matter what we do once we get in front of the judge.

I myself have made about a dozen appearances in family court. I have sued and I have been sued. In California, a dozen appearances in family court means another dozen appearances in mandatory mediation (a little room where an unelected judge sits in civilian clothes and tries to make you think you are not on trial). So, all told, I have French braided my hair and put on a "dry clean–only" outfit to sit in front of a stranger who would make decisions about my daughter's life a total of twenty-four times. In these seemingly unreal situations I've tried every approach I have ever heard of. I've tried the businesswoman look; I've tried the New Age professional look; I've tried the soccer mom look; I've tried being a doormat; I've tried being assertive; I've tried being weepy; I've even tried being aggressive; I've tried talking about "the child's best interest"; I've tried framing my comments around *my* best interest. Hell, girlfriends, I've tried witchcraft.

I tell you all of this not because I want to discourage you, but because I don't want you to get caught in the "I should have said . . ." vortex. I've had plenty of opportunities to say exactly what I "should have said . . ." the last time, and it hasn't done me a damn bit of good. Like most women, I discovered the hard way that the universe of family court is filled with, as Christopher Darden and many others have noted, "conflicts of interest, webs of politics, and the inbred, still-male-dominated world of lawyers and judges." Many of these folks profit off women's and children's misery, and because the Supreme Court hardly ever hears family law cases, even if our constitutional rights are violated, we often have no recourse.

Twenty-four attempts to make whichever social worker or judge or even lawyer I was talking to "get it" have taught me a little something: People who "get it" hardly ever work for family court. All my talking has left me feeling like Utah Philips trying to communicate with a Republican. It's "like trying to talk to a refrigerator," he says. "The light goes on, the light goes off, it's not going to do anything that's not built into it."

Sure, my soccer-mom-in-Neiman-Marcus look worked better than the New Age professional getup; my assertive-yet-teary-eyed approach made a better impression than my empowered-and-aggressive one; and framing my comments around "the child's best interest" worked a hell of a lot better than inviting the mediator to join my coven. But all of these attempts got me, essentially, the same response. If my ex wanted more time with our daughter, he got it. And if he didn't pay his child support, no one really cared. See, not only do people who work for family court fail to "get it," but even the ones who bear uncanny resemblances to my radical feminist friends only have about three conclusions built into them. There's "She's crazy and he's concerned," "She's hysterical and he's doing his best under stressful circumstances," and there's "She needs therapy and he needs more freedom and fewer bills to pay."

So what little gems of wisdom can I offer you if you're on your way to family court? Well . . .

- See if you can get screwed on your own terms—consult with an attorney, try to draft an agreement you can live with, and get your ex to sign it. I realize this is easier said than done, but as one family lawyer puts it, "Mom has the most power one time and one time only—*before* they ever walk into that courtroom. Once dad sees what really goes on in there, he'll be holding all the cards."

- If you do get a court and/or mediation date, *show up*. It's true that you won't have to watch yourself get screwed if you're not there, but just take this one on faith: If you ain't there, they'll take you for everything you've got—and more.

- In court and in mediation, try to kiss some serious butt. Be assertive and stand up for what you think is best for the kids, but *please* pretend to respect the judge, mediator, and/or anyone with any power.

- Bring copies of any applicable documents (i.e., proof of your income, proof of your major expenses, restraining orders, police reports, etc.).

- If you do try witchcraft, don't bring much paraphernalia with you. It's all right if your John the Conqueror root anointed with peppermint oil drops onto the floor (everyone will just think you were carrying around an old piece of shit), but dropping a doll full of pins and a large metal pentagram . . . well, it's just not the look we're going for.

- Don't call anyone a "big fat hairy loser who never could get it up anyway!" At least not out loud.

- Phrase your comments around "the child's best interest." Refer to the kids as "ours" rather than "mine."

- Remember: You are not crazy. You are stuck in a crazy system.

- Try to remain calm and businesslike.

- Remember to breathe.

- Keep both feet on the courtroom floor and know that the earth beneath it will hold you up.

Helping Our Kids Through

My friend Julia recently gave me a fabulous cartoon clipped from *The New Yorker*. A mama fish is telling her young "It's a very sad story, honey. I'm a single parent because I devoured your father." The little fishy looks slightly horrified, but one gets the feeling he'll be all right.

During family breakup, as during any other trauma, when the last thing we need is for our kids to get crabby, weird, extra needy, more vulnerable, aggressive, weepy, or whatever, that's just what they do. All of this is a normal response to what's going on. So try to be compassionate and help them out when you can. Cut them some slack, and they'll come back around in time.

Children can survive just about anything as long as they are told the truth about what is going on without feeling pressured to "take sides," but it's important to tell our kids a truth that is well thought out and age appropriate. The revelation, for example, that "mom and dad don't love each other anymore" begs the immediate, often unspoken response, "And when will you stop loving me?"

Kids need to know that there are different kinds of love and different kinds of commitments.

We can't control what our children's other parent does, but we can do our best to be a stable, supportive force in their lives. Most people I know who feel they got royally screwed by their parents' divorce got a load of crap from *both* sides. Here are some of my personal guidelines for dealing with my daughter and her dad. Yours might look a little different, but I think these are pretty basic:

- Tell the truth.

- Deal with issues as they arise.

- Respect my kid's relationship with her dad, regardless.

- Be as cordial to him as I can.

- Rant to friends and acquaintances when I'm pissed off, not to my kid.

- Assure my kid that whatever's up, it's not her fault and not her job to worry about.

- Refrain from making judging or nasty comments—even under my breath.

- Keep legal and court issues to myself whenever possible.

- Read children's books about nontraditional families; make sure there are other nontraditional families in my kid's life.

- Be a stable force in my kid's life.

- Keep absolutely every promise made.

At first, telling the truth and not dissing your kid's other parent might seem mutually exclusive, but they aren't. We will have many opportunities in our kids' lives to support their feelings, even when we don't share them. And family breakup is as good a time as any to get started. Basically, if our kids say they miss their other parent—or whatever—we have two choices. We can say "Why would you miss a brainless, gutless dork like that?" or we can affirm their feelings by saying something like "It must be hard having us live in different homes now." No matter what a brainless, gutless dork your ex may be, if you've ever been a kid, you know which answer is cooler.

If we run into our lawyer in line at the grocery store, we can simply introduce our child to them as "one of the people who is helping your dad and me work our schedules out."

If we have divorced because of family violence, we can say something like "Dad is having a lot of problems with anger and hitting. It is not our fault. And it is safer for us not to live with him anymore."

When a breakup is under way, it's often unclear what the eventual visitation schedule with look like. We can be honest about that too. We can say "We don't know how often you will see your dad yet, but we are trying to work it out as quickly as we can."

These are truths.

I don't mean to say that we have to protect the other parent. Our children may well feel abandoned or hurt by mom or dad. But we can support their feelings of betrayal without fueling them with our own. As my friend Amrita says, "When I hear something that really upsets me, I have to bite my tongue and just ask my son, 'How do you feel about that?'"

We also don't necessarily need to hide our feelings of disappointment and rage, as long as we don't direct them at our kids. One friend was so pissed off at her ex when he ran off with another woman, she beat her furniture every day for three years. Her children, eventually, got used to it. They would come home from school with friends, who would inevitably ask what was going on, and they just said, "Oh, that's my mom beating my dad."

Pulling Through

"I just took the kids to a baby-sitter and went out to see a punk band. Everyone in the audience was screaming like they wanted to kill someone, so I didn't feel out of place. Afterward I walked home real slow to chill out and stopped at a 7-Eleven to pick up some herbal tea."   —Yvette, twenty-four

"I was so stressed out I wasn't even sure I could put a sentence together. I just tried to remember that attorneys and judges and courts—none of those things are real. I imagined this tube of blue light running through my body and connecting me to the earth, and it helped."   —Lillianne, forty-one

"Every day I just told myself, 'All I have to deal with is today. Can I make it through today without blowing up at the kids? Can I keep my shit together at this one appointment? Can I pay for this one massage? Can I deal with this challenge in a way that I'll be proud of later?' Sometimes the big picture is just too big."
                                      —Kim, thirty-five

"My divorce got so violent and ugly so fast. I went to stay with my parents but they just said, 'Well, if he did all these horrible things, you must have driven him to it.' It took all my energy to find people who would help me say 'No, this is not my fault.' But I found those people. And I just refused to sink."   —Maria, thirty

The Long Haul

We all know that family breakup is difficult and messy. But often it turns out to be a good thing. We wouldn't put ourselves through all the storming hell if there wasn't some prize—some kind of spring—at the end of the long, long winter. We have a new family structure, our home is different. It's not broken, we realize, it's just different. Often we are freer, happier, and smarter for our troubles. Whatever it was in the relationship that was bogging us down and holding us back, whatever it was that we fought so hard to transform, has changed.

After a sweeping hill fire in Oakland a few years back, I saw a woman on the news standing in the ashes of her former home, holding a charred bowl. "I lost everything," she was saying, but by the look on her face I could tell it was a lie. "We lost all of our things. I lost the dissertation I had been working on for ten years. There is no other copy. But, look," she said, patting her chest and then pointing to some other family members who were standing by the chimney that was once connected to a house. "We're alive. And look," she said, turning to point at something behind her before the newscaster butted in. She was motioning toward the trees still standing a short distance up the hill or at some portion of the sky. I imagined she was trying to show off something beautiful she could see from her property now that there were no structures blocking the view.

Rebel Mom

Divorcing Gracefully

Opal Palmer Adisa, writer-professor mama,
author of It Begins with Tears *and other novels*

I know you've been divorcing for almost a year, but you never seem like you are falling apart. Perhaps you have some advice about divorcing gracefully?

On the one hand it's true that I haven't fallen apart, but I took this year off work. I'd been working very hard for ten years, so I took the time off for this transition—for myself and for my kids.

Divorce felt like a failure to me. And my kids are still very shaken by it. Marriage was something I wanted for my kids. It was something I invested a lot of time in. I think initially when we separated, I survived by working. My coping mechanism on one level was to pretend like it wasn't happening. I put it aside. I had to finish the semester, and I couldn't fall apart in front of my students. They depended on me. My kids depended on me too.

A lot of people say you shouldn't be angry, but I think that's bullshit. If you've invested time in the marriage, if you thought it was going to last a lifetime, if you thought you were going to be able to give your children that stability, then you have to feel the anger, the disappointment, the sense of failure. Something traumatic has happened. Divorce is the number-two major trauma people experience, next to the death of a loved one.

Much later one can put it aside, but during the summer I had to acknowledge that sense of rage, of betrayal, of being tricked. I almost could never say my ex-husband's name without it being followed by "motherfucker," and I usually do not swear.

People told me it would take three or four years to get over that anger, and I thought, "Oh, no. I don't have another four years to invest in this." So, in my typical expedient manner, I went into it and felt the full force of my rage. If I had suppressed that, it would have taken me much longer to get to a peaceful and accepting place.

How did you help your kids through that time?

Oh, I was saved. My mom took the kids for two months, so they were outside the fighting range. They were outside my uproar. My mother knew, because she was divorced. She offered to take them in her home in Jamaica for two months of the summer. By the time I went to get them in August, they were much different kids. Being outside the firing range, being there with my mother, being able to go to the beach helped them immeasurably.

And by August, most of my anger was gone. It had been replaced with sadness, a kind of melancholy, the part where you say "Where did it go wrong?" and "How come I could fix it before and I couldn't fix it this time?"

So, in that second phase, I got us all into therapy. I had had such a busy life schedule that I knew I needed not to work and I needed to spend more time with them. And more time with myself. I was a single mom now, and in the marriage I had been fortunate that my husband really did his share, so suddenly everything was up to me. That seemed at first overwhelming. We have been fooled by the feminist movement that says women can do it all themselves, but they can't.

When I was little in Jamaica, my mother always had domestic help, so being totally on my own felt crazy. The clothes bin is piled with clothes, I don't iron anything, the floor doesn't get mopped. Before, that would have been unheard of, but I've had to prioritize. And most days I'd much rather go to the park than mop the floor.

Also, being forty-two and reaching this place I hadn't prepared for. I had to step back and ask, "Where do I go with my life?"

Did you guys have a hard time working out custody issues?

Oh, yes. There was a tremendous battle over custody. Part of that was because we were still so angry at each other. The kids are very important to me, and they are very important to him. But on some level, they were the only thing we could fight over.

How do you balance being honest with your kids and not being too honest . . .

I didn't want to lie. I didn't like him, so I wasn't going to pretend that I liked him. I felt like I no longer knew him; as if I'd never truly known him. But I emphasized to the children that my relationship with their dad is different from their relationship with him. I said, "You can love your Baba and have a wonderful time with him, I just don't want to be with him."

Is the custody question settled now?

We have joint custody, but I am the primary custodian. They are with him every other weekend and one night a week for dinner.

At first I hated that. There was this inertia, and I did almost nothing when they were gone, but I have grown to look forward to their weekends away. I can clean the house. I can get some time to myself. I can work. But I do worry about how all of this will affect their sense of place, their sense of stability.

I am disturbed by the whole notion that it is parents who get divorced, not children. That's not true. They get divorced from a lifestyle that they had invested in too. Most of us by choice wouldn't want to be shuttled back and forth between two houses.

I resent that there are now major parts of their lives that I am not a part of. Things can happen when they are with him that I will never know about. The transitions are hard too. They are with him Friday through Monday, so on those Tuesdays when they return, I do not place any demands on them. We just hang out and have fun.

Is there a positive side to divorce?

For someone like me, it has been an opportunity to stop and reassess my life, and what I want to do with my life, and what kind of life I want for my kids. I was raised middle class, and my husband was raised working class. What I would think of as necessities, he would call "spoiling." So some of the things I used to have to negotiate, I can just do now. While you have to rely fully on yourself as a single mom, you can also do what you want with your kids. I also really enjoy having my own life. I like having my own room. The kids crawl into my bed at various times during the night, and that feels natural to me. I think I am a better mother now. I am more the mother I wanted to be. And I have a built-in break every other weekend.

We'd all rather avoid all the traumas that life throws in our paths. But once we pull through, once we realize that we will survive, few of us would go back and alter the past. When something ends, after all, something new begins. It always does.

"New seed is faithful," says Clarissa Pinkola Estés. "It roots deepest in the places that are most empty." So have faith, and be proud of all that you have survived. It's part of who you are.

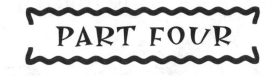

PART FOUR

BECOMING THE MAMA YOU ARE

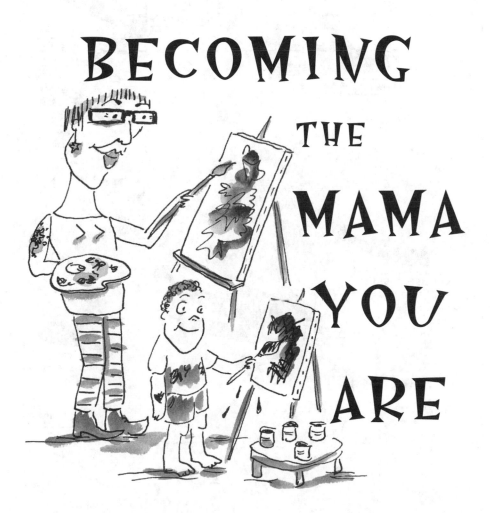

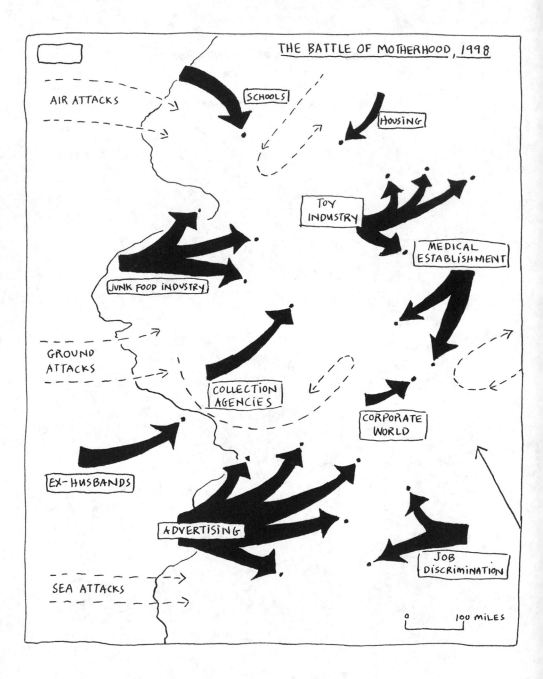

Chapter 12

Guerrilla Mothering

Never accept an expert's opinion if it violates your own because the experts can change their minds. Obedience to your own truth is the only safe ground to stand on, for only your own explanations will be defensible in court someday.

—*Mary Kay Blakely*

A guerrilla soldier always has great revolutionary vision but rarely the military training to back it up. The guns are stacked against her. She's outnumbered. And all logic says she doesn't have a chance in hell.

So why is it that nothing strikes fear in the heart of a general like the thought of confronting some ragtag guerrilla warrior in the unknown jungle? Simple: The guerrilla soldier is fighting from her heart, she's not simply "following orders." She knows the territory. She doesn't play by the rules. Sometimes she retreats, but she never surrenders.

Over the years, I have noticed that the mamas who seem to survive with their spirit and their sense of humor intact aren't necessarily the ones with the most money or the biggest husbands or the best recipes for marshmallow squares—they are the ones who approach motherhood like guerrilla soldiers defending their homelands. They're not paranoid. They know how to chill. But when they hear an enemy approaching, they're always ready.

What do our enemies look like? The danger we often feel lurking around the corner takes many forms. There are criminals, bullies, nervous breakdowns, ex-husbands, collection agents, monsters real and imagined. As if those weren't enough, we often find even more adversaries within the institutions where we go for help. We find them in the medical establishment, in the school system, in the toy and advertising industries, in the corporate work world, in the social services department, and in the court system. We are up against a whole culture that teaches mothers to be obedient to all of these institutions; to make cookies when we should be making revolutions; to work double shifts when we should be kicking back with our kids; to follow an "expert's" advice when we should be following our hearts.

Guerrillas—or "resistance fighters"—are all of those "lightly armed irregulars operating behind enemy lines," according to my *Penguin Encyclopedia of Modern Warfare*. And when our lives as moms feel like battlefields, I think we can all relate to those lightly armed irregulars. After all, resistance—as Alice Walker has pointed out—is the secret of joy. And, perhaps, the secret of motherhood.

A Place Called Tenacity

I don't think there is a "mothering instinct" built into us when it comes to things like figuring out how to feed our new babies, but the urge to protect our kids is both fierce and instinctual. Take the kickboxer Ramona Gatto. She had quit the sport by the time she had her daughter, but she came out of retirement with a new determination as a mom. She soon learned to fight, she once told an interviewer, not just to best an opponent, but as if "this person was taking food out of my child's mouth." With the energy she summoned with that thought, she became a world champion.

"Motherhood is a radicalizing experience," one veteran mom assures me. And it is. It always is. As mothers, we find ourselves caring so much more deeply about everything that happens in the world, and in our lives, because everything, whether we like it or not, relates to *our* children. There are times when it feels like we will never make it across all the minefields of mama hatred and child unfriendliness that we have to traverse to get the job, or the court order, or the peace of mind, or whatever elixir we feel we need to survive. But we go for it anyway.

One friend found herself totally distressed when her daughter turned one and started to walk. She sent me an E-mail saying "I could always protect my baby and control her environment so that she would be safe. Can I still do that?"

"Motherhood isn't just a series of contractions, it's a state of mind," Erma Bombeck wrote. "From the moment we know life is inside us, we feel a responsibility to protect and defend that human being. It's a promise we can't keep." But we try. We try passionately.

When Linda, a twenty-one-year-old lesbian mom, heard her son's teacher tell him that kids could "only have one mom," she firmly told the teacher otherwise and immediately set up a gay and lesbian awareness workshop for the preschool's staff.

When my friend Gwen got a notice from the sheriff's department that she and her four children had to vacate the county property where they had been camping in an old school bus, she rallied a few community members to help her fight the officials. She outright refused to leave the property until the county agreed to find her some affordable housing. The place she finally moved into was a little run-down, but it worked.

When one friend was told by her son's teacher that he would be held back in first grade because he had a different way of learning from many of his classmates, she worked with the school for a while, but when she found it totally lacking, she set up a home school co-op.

When a mama I interviewed was fighting a particularly heinous and abusive ex-husband in family court, her lawyers told her that she "just had to wait until he hits the child" before she could get visitation stopped, so she went guerrilla too. Her lawyers were right about the court system, but wrong about what she had to do. Instead of waiting for a tragedy, this mama got her four-year-old on a black-belt track in karate and got the hell out of family court.

Before we have children, it's almost always better to stay and fight for what we believe in. But once we have little ones depending on us, we have to weigh the costs. Sometimes we have to leave a protest when the riot cops arrive on the scene. This is not surrender. We just give up a little territory and create our own no-fire zones. Then we can come back, tell our stories, and fight the battles without putting our children in any extra danger.

Don't Shoot

Do you remember Ellie Nesler? She was the northern California mom who shot and killed the man accused of molesting her son. She just walked into the courtroom and shot him. She was, of course, celebrated as a great mama hero by many—we can all relate to her instinct—but she went to jail anyway—for four long years.

When the enemy is a person—someone who harms our kids—our instinct is to shoot first and ask questions later, but our children need us alive. And they need us out of jail.

For those of us who feel ambivalent, if not downright contemptuous, of our legal system, it can be hard to hand over our power. As my sister says, "You know you're desperate when you have to ally yourself with the cops." But we do. Sometimes we do. In this crazy land of motherhood that can at times feel like a war zone, the battle lines are constantly shifting, and we find ourselves behind enemy lines more often than not, standing next to people we never thought we'd come anywhere near.

Protection and Overprotection

Fortunately, most of us will never know exactly how Ellie Nesler felt as she lifted her gun, but we do know the milder dilemmas of protection and overprotection. No matter how fiercely we want to protect our kids, from the first labor pains we know that parenting is the slow process of letting go. When do we trust our instincts to protect and when do we let go and have faith?

For example, "When do I start letting my daughter play outside without a grown-up watching?" my friend Cynthia asks. Not at one, certainly. Probably not at two. At three or four if we feel that we live in a safe place and there are older children around? At twelve? How long do we stay and fight in family court? In our children's school? On the county's property? These are decisions we all have to make when they present themselves to us. And—I am sorry to say—there is no formula. There is only instinct and faith. When kids weren't allowed to do all the things I was when I was a little, my mother called them "overprotected." Perhaps they were, but all of these choices are personal, individual matters that we each have to weigh for ourselves and our children.

Phavia Kujichagulia, a griot and author of *Recognizing and Resolving Racism*, says that from the time her kids were born, she knew she could not protect them—only teach them. "If you live near a cactus, you can't move the cactus," she once told an interviewer for *Hip Mama*. "When they were growing up I had to get them to understand what was safe and what wasn't." She had to let them prick their fingers sometimes, let a little blood flow—not much—but like all of our children, they had to learn some lessons on their own.

"Although guerrillas have won total successes," my *Encyclopedia of Modern Warfare* tells me, the vast majority of us have been "contained in struggles which continue for years."

This doesn't mean that we shouldn't continue to, as they say, fight the good fight. It just means that we need to relax, make do, and enjoy ourselves along the way.

Taking Leave

One of my first childhood memories is a cover of *Ms.* magazine that pictured a many-armed goddess-woman doing everything at once. I'm not sure if it was supposed to represent oppression or liberation. Often it feels like both.

When I first became a mom, I sometimes felt judged by my older feminist friends who seemed to be saying "What? We did all of this work and you just go get yourself knocked up? You want to be just a mother?" But for me there was never any concept of being "just a mother."

I always had the sense that I had many arms. Certainly I had to remember to take care of my own soul, not to do everything at once all of the time, not to get too tired and stressed out. But I have always known that, when necessary, I could use as many of my arms as a situation required.

So what was this about "just a mother"?

Over the years, I think I have begun to understand. And I have come to appreciate my feminist mothers' initial concern. The institution of motherhood *has* been used to oppress us. As feminist mothers, we are irregulars operating behind enemy lines. But the reaction I felt as judgment was more like "Holy shit, wait until you are ready." Not necessarily "ready" as in old enough, but wait until you are strong enough within yourself not to get totally creamed by the bullshit society has in store for you once they see you as "just a mother." Once they expect you to be obedient to everything but your own heart.

But ready or not, I became a mother, as you did. And when we start to feel like maybe we aren't quite strong enough within ourselves, we have to retreat. We have to step back, if not from the philosophical dilemmas of motherhood, then at least from the practical ones.

"Every person deserves a day away in which no problems are confronted, no solutions searched for," Maya Angelou wrote in *Wouldn't Take Nothing for My Journey Now*. And even the most committed guerrilla mother has to agree. We need leave days to, as my friend Jackie says, "do nothing but shop at The Gap or walk four miles or make voodoo dolls of our ex-boyfriends or get laid."

We need leave days to kick back, to say "I did what I could and I deserve a beer," as Ani DiFranco puts it.

"I've been doing all this girly stuff lately," my friend Alana told me the other day, with just the slightest tinge of guilt in her voice. "I went and got my nails done last week, and then I got a tiny tattoo on my hand yesterday," she went on. "I've gotta get these shoes for my kids, but I've gotta do some shit for myself. I shouldn't feel guilty, should I?"

"Do their feet hurt?" I asked.

"No."

So, no. She shouldn't feel guilty. Not even the slightest little bit. But it can be hard to remember to take time out from just being "mommy," especially when we know our kids could always use one more pair of shoes, a bigger trike, or some organic apple juice instead of the frozen stuff.

"You won't be doing your kids any favors by being a martyr," I reminded her.

Whenever I ride in an airplane and hear the old emergency procedures drill, I worry that in a panic I wouldn't be able to follow the steward's instructions to "secure your own oxygen mask before assisting young children." But the airline folks are right. Sometimes we can't be any help to our children if we haven't taken care of ourselves.

In a "Mother's Day Maxim" the poet Opal Palmer Adisa once sent me, she suggested being selfish for the day. She wrote:

> do not answer to the words: mother, mommie,
> mom or any of those ghastly terms that have
> canceled out your own name.

My first thought, of course, was "I can't do that!" my daughter *needs* me. But my daughter doesn't need me all day every day. I could, and I did, take some time to myself.

We all need time spent in solitude. We also need to get out with other moms, or with childless girlfriends, and just have fun. We need a "girls' night out" every now and again.

We need to have romantic and sexual lives too. We need to get out with our partners or, if we are single, feel free to have lovers without having to parade each of them in front of our kids. It might be easier to rent a video and spend every Saturday night with the baby, but after the first weeks or months of parenthood, Blockbuster just doesn't cut it.

One married mama I know actually takes her own parents with her on vacations. The couple doesn't want to leave the kids at home, but they need the built-in baby-sitting services her parents can provide— it's cheaper than an au pair, after all.

As our kids grow, their lives become more complex too—with preschool and elementary schedules, teams, classes, and appointments of all kinds. Once we've learned how to take care of ourselves, we need time out with our kids too.

Every once in a while, I just let Maia stay home from school, and we both wear sweats and do whatever we please. A child counselor I once talked to even assured me that loosening up the rules actually would make Maia less likely to break them when I didn't want her to.

When I was six, it snowed in the California suburb where we lived. Given the mild climate, this was literally a once-in-a-lifetime event, so my mother let my sister and I "play hooky." We got in a little trouble when we went onto the schoolyard to build a snowman, but we managed to get away from the screaming principal and run home to mom, who was, at least for the day, on our side of the battle line. But why wait for a blizzard in California to feel okay about a little harmless truancy?

Rebel Mom

Susie Sexpert: Lightly Armed & Irregular

Susie Bright, sex-positive feminist mama; author,
Susie Bright's Sexwise, Sexual State of the Union,
and other books

First things first: What's your personal formula for teaching your kid about sex?

My commandments so far are

Thou shalt not lie.

Thou shalt not be a hypocrite.

- Tell your children the names for their genitals. A two-year-old can pronounce "clitoris," and she needs to know what the differences are between her vagina, her pee-hole (urethra), her anus, her vulva (or any cute name you want to call it), and her clit. She needs to know, just like little boys, that these are the parts of her body involved in making babies and that they are also a source of special physical pleasure—she'll find out sooner or later, and you don't want her to wonder if she's the only one!

- Be nonchalant and supportive about masturbation.

- Give your kid the same privacy you would like for yourself. Don't bust into their rooms, demand they tell you their fantasies and dreams, insist on inspecting every little thing. Show that you can really listen and feel compassion for their concerns when they bring up *any* topic, so when they bring up sexual questions or fears, they'll trust you not to go berserk.

- Tell them when they are old enough about all the religious prohibitions about sexuality, so they can understand why there are so many "rules" about sexual behavior. If you are a faith-observing person who is open-minded about sex, explain to them that those things are compatible to you, that you don't have to forsake your beliefs for sex, or vice versa. I'm part of a multigeneration of Catholic girls who grew up associating hell and punishment and Satan with sexual feelings. Don't go there!

We were talking the other day about your traditional-looking family situation. You've got the big house with the almost-picket fence. You've got the big man . . .

I actually want to build a wall out of rocks and driftwood and flowering bushes where that broken old fence is now. It's a very romantic fantasy, this house. It's like my own private fairy tale just living here. I grew up in apartments with cottage-cheese ceilings and no-children rules that my mother did God-knows-what to get an exception for us. I had to present myself as very obedient and quiet, which I was.

I don't have any family role models for marriage or long-lasting relationships. In fact, I am attending my first real wedding at age thirty-nine, this very April. My live-in partner and I have gotten where we are today through the weirdest route. We were in love with other people when we first started seeing each other . . . other people who weren't in love with us. We've never been monogamous, we're both bisexual, and we are philosophically twins about sexuality. Living together wise, we're just strangely compatible. I didn't know that until we tried it a year ago. I've known him for seven years. Our love and trust for each other grew through trials and tribulations, that's for sure. His relationship with Aretha, my daughter, grew slowly. Nothing happened because of wild declarations or promises. I am such an impulsive, charge-ahead person that this is more shocking than it might be for other people.

It's good to have a home you love. It's good to have people who love you no matter what. It's good to have a lover you can confide in and who you trust with your sexual imagination and disposition. It's good to have a chosen family that works out, because man, the one you're born into may have all the seams ripped out before you know it.

Jon is unique to me, just like Aretha, but truth be told, there are a few other people in my life I couldn't live without. It's just that they don't presently live in the same house as me. But we love each other and depend on each other just as fiercely. I feel like they get over-looked when people ask me about my partner and kid. I believe in a tribe loyalty, I guess. I wish I could have a ceremony that honors all our relationships with one another, not just one lover.

Tell me more about your extended chosen family. Did you ever feel a sense of isolation as a mama, or was your community pretty well established before you got pregnant?

No, I lived alone with Aretha for the first four years, and many times I lost my temper at her and wanted to go crazy, which would have been alleviated by another grown-up being there. Other times I was just lonely and felt like I couldn't cope with work and home stuff simultaneously. Nothing unusual, just the typical mom grind. I think that even women with installed husbands and in-laws find themselves holding the bag many times.

Yeah. What do you do to relax and mellow out when you think you are becoming a crazed mama?

Crawl into bed. Close the door and don't let anyone in. Read stupid celebrity magazines and get engrossed in evening gowns. Television, web surfing, novel reading, massage, bathtub soaking—those are other favorites. Once last spring I climbed up high into an oak tree and didn't come down for several hours.

There are no rules when it comes to resistance, but, in hopes of finding some guidelines, I recently I went looking for a guide to guerrilla warfare. I didn't find what I was looking for, so, as usual, I ended up having to take what guidance I could get from other moms and ad-lib the rest. Here's what I came up with:

- Eat well.
- Rest well.
- Be obedient to your own truth.
- Protect by teaching.
- Love strongly.
- Listen thoughtfully.
- Choose your battles carefully.
- Trust your intuition.
- Think before you shoot.
- Use your weapons: your voice, your mind, and your heart.
- Know your allies, and call on them often.
- Remember to climb up into an oak tree every now and again.

All logic says we don't have a chance in hell—but I think we know better than that.

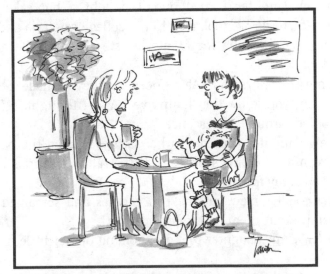

"Kids are a pain in the ass, but definitely a worthwhile, fulfilling pain in the ass."

Chapter 13

Imperfectly

~~~~~~~~~~~~~~~~

There seemed to be several avenues open to me: (a) take myself seriously and end up drinking gin before the school bus left; (b) take the children seriously and end up drinking gin before the school bus left; (c) admit to the fear and frustration and have a good time with it.
— *Erma Bombeck*

When my daughter turned one, I bought a big cake with a bounced check. We took it in to my college cafeteria and as I lit the candle, she took the first tentative steps of her life across a smooth, dark floor.

One of my professors said, "Aaw, one. Once they've made it through that first year, you know they'll survive." And I thought, "Naw, she still has to live through adolescence."

When my daughter turned two her father crashed the party and sprayed green foam-string stuff all over the red decorations I'd carefully hung with my friends.

An older toddler blew out the two candles and screamed out in anger when we relit them for the birthday girl.

"Two is this," my daughter told me, holding up her little fingers in a peace sign.

When my daughter turned three, she had been waiting for the day as long as she could remember. "Am I going to be big when I am three?" she had asked me again and again and I had said "Yes."

"Big up over the ceiling?" she had asked, and I nodded and smiled and never thought much about the question.

But when she blew out her three candles, instinctively jerked backward from the shock of the cheer, and paused, she burst into tears. She'd thought she'd grow suddenly—like Alice—big up over the ceiling. And she was still small.

When my daughter turned four I scarcely caught glimpses of her at the huge party we'd scheduled around daddy visits. I'd followed my own mother's warning that "the other kids will feel soooo left out" and invited my daughter's thirty preschool classmates and twelve neighbor kids.

One girl showed up with two moms and my daughter was jealous. "She has two moms, but soon I'm going to have three moms and I'm going to be the winner," she insisted.

A trial-size bottle of ibuprofen did nothing for my headache, and my daughter passed out from exhaustion before she opened her last present.

When my daughter turned five, the sounds of Discovery Zone Fun Center were deafening. My pockets were empty after paying ten kids' way into the zone and spending countless quarters on games, and she was beside herself with excitement. But she was waiting. There was one child who received the bright clown invitation, who promised to come, who she hadn't seen in almost a year. And she waited all through the pizza and ice cream and arcade games and jumping into those seas of plastic balls and opening present after awesome present, asking every few minutes, "But where is *he*?" And I didn't know.

When my daughter turned six she worried she'd have to do more homework. She asked if she'd ever be a baby again. "When will I be a teenager?" she wanted to know. Almost halfway there.

And as I stirred the cake batter—the first time I'd baked in almost two years—it occurred to me that I could not even begin to imagine what my late teens and early twenties would have been like without her all-encompassing energy, her croons of "I love you, sweet mama," her shouts of "I'll never love you again, funky mama," her dreams of big and small.

My daughter is seven now—just turned a few weeks ago—and we have retreated to the high desert of northern New Mexico. I have a meeting here, but we are planning to stay away an extra week.

Our first night out is disorienting. It is so quiet at the Ghost Ranch where we are staying, Maia and I think we can hear the snow falling onto the red earth. She scoops up a handful, packs it tightly, and pegs me right between the eyes.

"I need a cup with a lid so I can take some snow back to California," Maia tells me. "If it melts on the way and then we put it in the freezer, will it be snow or ice?"

"Ice," I tell her, and she is disappointed.

As we are unpacking our pajamas, yesterday's "to-do" list that somehow ended up in my bag falls to the floor. Glancing over it, I have to laugh:

- Do dishes
- Write column
- Help Maia start science project
- Cancel therapy
- Buy snowsuit for Maia
- Find substitute for Hip Mama radio show
- Update zine subscriber list
- Finish book
- Do laundry
- Take out garbage

I exhale and let the last of my vacation guilt melt away. I cannot be that many-armed goddess all of the time. We deserve a little time in high desert where we can hear the snow falling onto the ground. We deserve a few days where there are no teachers, no mandatory science projects, no bill collectors, no laundry, no deadlines. A few days when we can laugh at our "to-do" lists and take on more realistic goals:

- Wake up
- Eat breakfast
- Play in the snow
- Go to the paleontology museum if we feel like it
- Wander

- Eat lunch
- Play some more . . .

In one of her diaries, Anaïs Nin wrote: "The presence of the young lightens the world and changes it from an oppressive, definitive, solidified one to a fluid, potentially marvelous, as-yet-to-be-created world." I know this is true, so I'm embarrassed to admit that I rarely stop and appreciate that fluidity, that as-yet-to-be-created world where I can laugh when Maia pegs me between the eyes with a snowball instead of thinking "Christ, not another damn thing coming at me."

I go to the meeting, but then we spend several more days at the ranch doing nothing much at all. On Saturday, we head over to Ojo Caliente, a natural hot spring, and we float in the mineral pools. Monday morning we are off again, this time to see some friends who live outside Santa Fe.

As we are driving slowly along the unpaved, unmarked New Mexico roads, Maia asks about the people we are going to see. They are the parents of a good friend of mine who died when I was a kid. I speak softly as I try to explain the girl's death. Her name was Jessica. She had cancer, had her leg amputated when we were in fifth grade, but got sick again and died when we were in seventh grade.

"But how did she *get* cancer?" Maia asks.

"We don't know," I tell her as I search my mind for an answer to her unasked question, *Could that happen to me?*

Sometimes I am at such a loss, mothering in this world where "There's so much cancer, so much plague," as Anne Lammot puts it. "There are so goddamn many child-snatchers, psychopaths. Republicans."

Often I have the answers to Maia's questions, or I can feign some sort of control. I tell Maia that if we learn self-defense, we will be able to fight off the psychopath. If we study economics and sociology, we can outlogic the Republicans. When we hear of car accidents, I promise to drive carefully. When we see poison berries at the edge of a path, I warn her not to eat them. When we make a wrong turn and get stuck in the snow, I stop, push the car out of danger, and make a U-turn. But now I am silent.

I want desperately to tell Maia, and myself, that nothing terrible could ever happen to us. I think to tell her something that I was once told as a kid: that God only gives us as much hardship as we can handle. But I decide to spare her the bizarre concept. I have spent too much of my life trying not to look like I could handle a great deal.

"Not very many children get cancer," I finally say. "Not very many at all." At least we have statistics on our side.

Maia smiles thoughtfully and turns back to looking for jackrabbits and the final landmark that will tell us we are headed in the right direction on this winding dirt road.

My own fears, however, are not so easily calmed.

I wish I could develop some kind of Zen mind around all of this. I wish I could teach Maia, with confidence, that "life is about not knowing, having to change, taking the moment and making the best of it, without knowing what is going to happen next," as Gilda Radner put it. "Delicious ambiguity."

But as we drive up into these snow-covered mountains, as we make a sharp right turn on the road that is supposed to be marked by a *"Camino Quien Sabe"* sign, as we drive toward the home of these friends, these parents who have survived my greatest fear—losing my daughter—I don't have any motherly wisdom to offer.

I grip the steering wheel tightly as our rental car slips a little on a patch of ice and the tires spin in the thick red mud. It's times like these when I think to myself, *Well, Ms. Hip Mama parenting expert, you've read all the books, you know you are supposed to be honest, you know you can talk about things without getting all wrapped up in your own fears, and yet . . . silence.*

"How do you know this is the right road?" Maia finally asks me.

"I don't," I have to admit. "There was no sign. But one way or another, I'm pretty sure we'll get there."

"Did you cry when Jessica died?" she wants to know.

"Yes," I tell her. "I cried. Everyone cried. When terrible things happen we have to cry. Things like that—getting cancer, dying young—we feel like they aren't supposed to happen, but sometimes they do. I don't think anything like that will happen to us, but, you know, that's why we have to watch for jackrabbits now. That's why it matters that the mountains are beautiful now. That's why we have to pay attention to the magic. And that's why it doesn't really matter if we take chances and make mistakes sometimes too. Because we don't know for sure what's going to happen in the future. I believe people's spirits live on even when their bodies stop working, though. What do you think?"

"I think this is the right road," she tells me. And we smile.

There is no doubt: This journey we are on as mothers is treacherous. Instead of clear road signs we get questions we don't know the answers to. The path is marked with joys and dangers, laughter and wrong turns, glorious views and insults of all kinds. There are days when I feel like I am God's gift to my daughter—the best mama anyone could hope to have. Other times I feel like I am mothering along an unmarked, unpaved road that winds along the edge of a steep desert cliff. A false turn of the wheel, an unexpected patch of ice in the road, or a momentary lapse of any kind could send us careening off the edge.

But as Maia grows older, more independent, and more capable of helping me watch for the landmarks along the way—as I grow more comfortable in my role as her witness and sometimes-helpful guide— I think, perhaps, I am beginning to relax into all of this delicious ambiguity. And the worst of my fears—along with my stretch marks—are fading.

We can be only who we are, after all, and we can give our children only what comes from our hearts. Every turn may take us a little farther from perfection, but when all is screamed and done, we will survive, I'm pretty sure. We will survive, Maia and I, you and your children, and all of us lightly armed irregulars and millennial families who are reinventing motherhood all over again. And we'll learn to relax, breathe, fight, and laugh a little along the way.

If there's one thing I've learned about mothering, it's that there are a million ways to raise good kids, and none of them is perfect.

"Give them that which truly comes from yourself, your doubts and contradictions," says Anilú Elías. "And, above all, enjoy it now. Their infancy will pass soon enough and later you'll miss everything but the quarrels. And like fireworks, you'll forget why they drove you so crazy."

SURVIVAL NOTES

Books

Pregnancy and Birth

Carroll Dunham and The Body Shop Team, *Mamatoto: A Celebration of Birth* (New York: Penguin, 1993).

Arlene Eisenberg, Heidi E. Murkoff, and Sandee E. Hathaway, B.S.N., *What to Expect When You're Expecting* (New York: Workman, 1991).

Ina May Gaskin, *Spiritual Midwifery* (Summertown, Tenn.: Book Publishing Co., 1977)

Barbara Harper, R.N., *Gentle Birth Choices* (Rochester, Vt: Healing Arts Press, 1997).

Sheila Kitzinger, *Your Baby, Your Way: Making Pregnancy Decisions and Birth Plans* (New York: Pantheon, 1987).

Randall Neustaedter, *The Immunization Decision* (Berkeley, Calif.: North Atlantic Books, 1993).

Margie Profet, *Protecting Your Baby-to-Be: Preventing Birth Defects in the First Trimester* (Reading, Mass.: Addison-Wesley, 1995).

Prudence and Sherill Tippins, *Two of Us Make a World: The Single Mother's Guide to Pregnancy, Childbirth, and the First Year* (New York: Henry Holt, 1996).

Mama Care

Maya Angelou, *Wouldn't Take Nothing for My Journey Now* (New York: Random House, 1993).

Boston Women's Health Book Collective, *The New Our Bodies, Ourselves* (New York: Simon & Schuster, 1992).

Robin Lim, *After the Baby's Birth . . . A Woman's Way to Wellness: A Complete Guide for Postpartum Women* (Berkeley, Calif.: Celestial Arts, 1991).

Clarissa Pinkola Estés, *Women Who Run With the Wolves* (New York: Ballantine Books, 1992).

Feminist and Antibias Child Rearing

Phavia Kujichagulia, *Recognizing and Resolving Racism: A Survival Guide for Humane Beings* (Oakland, Calif.: A. Wisdom Company, 1995).

Dr. Barbara Mackoff, *Growing a Girl: Seven Strategies for Raising a Strong, Spirited Daughter* (New York: Dell, 1996).

Mary Pipher, *Reviving Ophelia: Saving the Selves of Adolescent Girls* (New York: Ballantine Books, 1994).

Maureen T. Reddy, ed., *Everyday Acts Against Racism: Raising Children in a Multiracial World* (Seattle, Wash.: Seal Press, 1996).

Dena Taylor, ed., *Feminist Parenting: Struggles, Triumphs & Comic Interludes* (Freedom, Calif.: Crossing Press, 1994).

Politics & "Family Values"

Mary Kay Blakely, *American Mom: Motherhood, Politics and Humble Pie* (Chapel Hill, N.C.: Algonquin Books, 1994).

Susie Bright, *Susie Bright's Sexual State of the Union* (New York: Simon & Schuster, 1997).

Shere Hite, *The Hite Report on the Family: Growing Up Under Patriarchy* (New York: Grove Press, 1995).

Judith Stacey, *In the Name of the Family: Rethinking Family Values in a Post-Modern Age* (Boston: Beacon Press, 1996).

Single Mamahood

Shoshana Alexander, *In Praise of Single Parents: Mothers and Fathers Embracing the Challenge* (Boston: Houghton Mifflin, 1994)

Andrea Engber and Leah Klungness, *The Complete Single Mother* (Holbrook, Mass.: Adams Publishing, 1995).

Anne Lamott, *Operating Instructions* (New York: Fawcett, 1994).

Divorce & Family Law

Lois Brenner and Robert Stein, *Getting Your Share: A Woman's Guide to Successful Divorce Strategies* (New York: Crown, 1989).

Phyllis Chesler, *Mothers on Trial* (Seattle, Wash.: Seal Press, 1987).

Maria Gil de Lamadrid, ed., *Lesbians Choosing Motherhood: Legal Implications of Donor Insemination and Co-Parenting* (San Francisco: National Center for Lesbian Rights, 1991).

Robin Leonard and Stephen Elias, *Nolo's Pocket Guide to Family and Divorce Law* (Berkeley, Calif.: Nolo Press, 1996).

Karen Winner, *Divorced from Justice: The Abuse of Women and Children by Divorce Lawyers and Judges* (New York: HarperCollins, 1996).

For Teenagers

Allison Abner and Linda Villarosa, *Finding Our Way: The Teen Girls' Survival Guide* (New York: HarperPerennial, 1995).

Shirley Arthur, *Surviving Teen Pregnancy: Your Choices, Dreams and Decisions* (Buena Park, Calif.: Morning Glory Press, 1991).

Spirituality, Meditation, and Relaxation

Zsuzsanna Budapest, *The Grandmother of Time* (New York: Harper & Row, 1989).

Jon Kabat-Zinn, *Wherever You Go, There You Are: Mindfulness Meditation in Everyday Life* (New York: Hyperion, 1994).

Hugh and Gayle Prather, *Spiritual Parenting: A Guide to Understanding and Nurturing the Heart of Your Child* (New York: Harmony Books, 1996).

Elaine St. James, *Simplify Your Life: 100 Ways to Slow Down and Enjoy the Things That Really Matter* (New York: Hyperion, 1994).

Luisah Teish, *Jambalaya: The Natural Women's Book of Personal Charms & Practical Rituals* (San Francisco: HarperSanFrancisco, 1985).

Marianne Williamson, *Illuminata: A Return to Prayer* (New York: Riverhead, 1995).

Work and Money

Jolie Godfrey, *Our Wildest Dreams: Women Making Money, Doing Good, Having Fun* (New York: Harper Business, 1993).

Eric Tyson, *Personal Finance for Dummie$s* (San Mateo, Calif.: IDG Books Worldwide, 1995).

Anne C. Weisberg and Carol A. Buckler, *Everything a Working Mother Needs to Know about Pregnancy Rights, Maternity Leave, and Making Her Career Work for Her* (New York: Main Street Books, Doubleday, 1994).

Music and Other Sounds

Ladyslipper
Women's music catalog
P.O. Box 3124
Durham, NC 27715
(800) 634-6044
http://www.ladyslipper.org

Sounds True
Transformational audio
(800) 333-9185

Zines, Newsletters, and Magazines

Feminism

Bust: The Only Zine that Lifts and Separates
$12 for four issues
P.O. Box 319, Ansonia Station
New York, NY 10023
e-mail: bust@aol.com

HUES: Hear Us Emerging Sisters
$12.95 for four issues
P.O. Box 7778
Ann Arbor, MI 48107-8226
telephone: (313) 971-0450

Ms.
$45 for six issues
Subscription Dept.
Box 57122
Boulder, CO 80321-7122
telephone: (800) 234-4486

SageWoman: Celebrating the Goddess in Every Woman
$18 for four issues
P.O. Box 641
Point Arena, CA 95468
telephone: (707) 882-2052
http://www.sagewoman.com

Lesbian Mothering

Mom's Apple Pie:
Newsletter of the Lavender
Families Resource Network
$15 for four issues

Lavender Families Resource Network
P.O. Box 21567
Seattle, WA 98111
telephone: (206) 325-2643

Life as a Mom

Hip Mama: The Parenting Zine
$12 to $20 (sliding scale, you decide how
much to pay) for four issues
P.O. Box 9097
Oakland, CA 94613
telephone: (800) 585-MAMA or (510) 658-4508
e-mail: hipmama@sirius.com
http://www.hipmama.com

**The Mother Is Me: An Alternative
Publication on the Motherhood Experience**
$15.95 for four issues
P.O. Box 5174
Dover, NH 03821
telephone: (800) 693-6852
http://members.aol.com/zoey455/index.html

Poverty

Welfare Mothers Voice
$12 for four issues
2711 W. Michigan
Milwaukee, WI 53208
telephone: (414) 342-6662

Pregnancy, Birth, and Breast Feeding

Birth Gazette
$30 for four issues
42, The Farm
Summertown, TN 38483
telephone: (615) 964-2472
e-mail: brthgzt@usit.net

The Compleat Mother: The Magazine
of Pregnancy, Birth and Breastfeeding
$12 for four issues
Box 209
Minot, ND 58702
telephone: (701) 852-2822

Mothering
$18.95 for four issues
P.O. Box 1690
Santa Fe, NM 87504
telephone: (800) 984-8116
e-mail: mother@ni.net

For Single Mamas

SingleMOTHER: The Newsletter of the
National Organization of Single Mothers
$15 for membership and subscription
Box 68
Midland, NC 28107
telephone: (704) 888-5437
http://www.parentsplace.com/readroom/nosm

Organizations
and Hot Lines

(Local chapters of many of these organizations
can be found in your local phone book)

Addiction Recovery

- Alcohol and Drug Helpline offers referrals to drug detox and rehabilitation programs: (800) 252-6465
- Alcoholics Anonymous Worldwide Services offers information and referrals to local recovery support groups: (212) 870-3400

Adoption

- National Adoption Hotline offers information for women starting the adoption process: (202) 328-1200

Childbirth and Maternal Health

- American College of Nurse-Midwives offers referrals to local midwives: (888) 643-9433
- ASPO-Lamaze offers childbirth education information and local referrals: (800) 368-4404
- Association of Labor Assistants and Childbirth Educators (ALACE) offers information and referrals: (617) 441-2500
- Hill Burton Hotline offers hospital and medical care referrals for low-income mamas: (800) 638-0742
- La Leche League offers information and support group referrals on breast feeding: (800) LA-LECHE
- National Association of Childbearing Centers offers referrals to birthing centers in your area. Send one dollar to NACC, 3123 Gottschall Rd., Perkionenville, PA 18074
- National Association of Postpartum Care Service offers referrals to nonmedical postpartum caregivers: (800) 45-DOULA
- National Organization of Circumcision Information Resource Centers offers information on circumcision and the movement to end it: (415) 454-5669
- National Center for Education in Child and Maternal Health offers pre- and postnatal health resources including information on circumcision and breast feeding: (202) 625-8400

- Planned Parenthood Federation of America offers pregnancy counseling, prenatal care, and referrals: (800) 230-PLAN
- The Bradley Method offers information and referrals for classes on childbirth: (800) 4-A-BIRTH
- The Farm Clinic in Summertown, Tennessee, offers referrals to local home birth practitioners: (615) 964-2293
- YWCA offers prenatal classes, support groups, domestic violence referral services, child care, etc. Check your phone book or call: (212) 614-2700

Child Care

- Child Care Aware offers help finding child care in your area: (800) 424-2246
- Child Care Law Center offers legal information about child care: (415) 495-5498

Death and Bereavement

- National Sudden Infant Death Syndrome Resource Center offers literature and support for grieving parents: (703) 821-8955
- Widowed Persons Service offers support group referrals: (800) 424-3410

Domestic Violence and Parental Kidnapping

IF YOU HAVE AN EMERGENCY CALL 911

- Child Find Mediation Program offers information and mediation for parents who have abducted children and for parents who have lost children to parental kidnapping: (800) A-WAY-OUT
- National Center for Missing and Exploited Children helps locate missing children: (800) 843-5678
- National Coalition Against Domestic Violence has literature and support group referrals: (303) 839-1852
- National Domestic Violence Hotline offers twenty-four-hour information and referrals for battered women: (800) 799-7233
- National Family Violence Hotline offers twenty-four-hour information and referrals for battered women: (800) 222-2000

Divorce and Family Law

- Academy of Family Mediators offers help finding a mediator: (617) 674-2663
- American Society of Appraisers offers help finding an appraiser: (800) 272-8258
- Appraisal Institute offers help finding an appraiser: (312) 335-4100
- Find Dad is a national child support collection agency that works on commission: (800) 729-6667
- Lavender Families Resource Network offers support, legal resources, and information for lesbian parents: (206) 325-2643
- NOW Legal Defense and Education Fund offers information and kits on divorce, child support, custody, family law, and discrimination issues: (212) 925-6635
- Society of Professionals in Dispute Resolution offers help finding a mediator: (202) 783-7277

Mental Health and Support Groups

- A Circle of Sisters offers support group referrals for women of African ancestry: (212) 459-4806
- Depression After Delivery offers referrals to support groups and other contacts for depressed mamas: (800) 944-4773
- Family Resource Coalition offers help and information on finding or starting support groups: (312) 341-0900
- National Clearinghouse on Family Support & Children's Mental Health offers information and referrals to local family therapists: (800) 628-1696
- National Mental Health Association offers referrals to local therapists: (703) 684-7722

Poverty

- Welfare Warriors offers support and help to low-income, women: (414) 342-6662
- Federal Information Center provides phone numbers for information on federal programs: (800) 688-9889
- Single Parent Resource Center offers help for poor, low-income and working single parents; homeless families; and women returning to the community from prison: (212) 951-7030

Acknowledgments

A giant banana split for Maia ("I am not a princess, I am a queen") Swift. You know it. And for all the other little queens and kings in our lives—you are most fabulous.

Major thanks to my agents, Madeleine Morel and Barbara Lowenstein; and to my awesome editor, Laurie Abkemeier.

And a round of Pete's Wicked Ale for all the lightly armed irregulars operating behind enemy lines: Julie, Ophira Edut, Wendy DeJong, the amazing Mary Kay, Mary Lawton, Julia, my family, Eva and Joe, Lynn, Tom, Spike, Jeni, Vanessa Graves, Shamama, Linda French, and the Hip Mama family, known and unknown.

Here's to always being "conservative America's worst nightmare."

Subscribe to Hip Mama

Subscribe to *Hip Mama: The Parenting Zine!* It's a quarterly full of information, news, essays, fiction, poetry, photography, and art for progressive families. Call (800) 585-MAMA or (510) 658-4508 for more information, or check us out on the web: www.hipmama.com.

For a four-issue subscription, send the amount between $12 and $20 you decide you can afford to:

Hip Mama
P.O. Box 9097
Oakland, CA 94613

Name_____

Address _____

City _____State _____Zip _____

Index

Abner, Allison, 39–40

Abortion, 28, 152

Abusive relationships, 37, 38
  see also Domestic violence

Academy of Family Mediators, 212

Addiction, 22, 23

Adisa, Opal Palmer, 225–28, 237

Adolescence, 111

Adoption, 16–17

Advertising, 116–17

After the Baby's Birth (Lim), 75

Agitated depression, 178

Alcohol, 22

Al-Kebu-Lan, 30

American College of Nurse-
  Midwives, 45, 47, 49

*American Journal of Public
  Health*, 48

American Psychiatric Association, 176

American Psychological
  Association, 37

American Society of Appraisers, 211

American Way of Birth, The
  (Mitford), 53, 133

Amniocentesis, 29, 44

Amniotic sac, rupturing, 57, 59

Anal sex, 25

Anemia, 29

Anesthesiologist, 48

Angelou, Maya, 115, 236

Anger, 98, 103
  in divorce, 225–26, 227

Anxiety disorders, 176

Appraisal Institute, 211

Appraiser(s), 211

Art, 183

Association of Labor
  Assistants, 47

At-Home Mom, 142

Attorney(s), 36, 207, 208, 209,
  216, 217
  in family court, 220

Autonomy, 102–3

Baby(ies), 68–84

Baby shower, 30

Backaches, 28

Bad Mom, 143

Bankruptcy, 200

Bathroom supplies, 31

Batterers, 34, 38, 113–14, 152–53
  custody of children, 35, 37

Bed(s), baby, 31

Bed-wetting, 95

Bergers, Glen, 83–84

Bigotry, 115-16

Birth attendant, 65

Birth Coach, 48

Birth control, 81–82

Birth defects, 29

Birth Gazette, 49, 81

Birth mothers, 17

Birth partner, 45, 59

Birth plan, 44, 48, 58–60, 65

Birthing centers, 45, 47, 52

Blakely, Mary Kay, 119–21, 197

Bleeding gums, 28

Blended families, 155, 156

Bloating, 24

Body Manipulations, 27

Body Shop, 54

Bombeck, Erma, 80, 233

Bonding, 45-46
  in nursing, 76

Bottle-feeding, 30

Bottles, 30

Bowles, Julie, 65–66

Bradley method, 46

Breast-feeding, 30, 59, 76–79, 93
  tips for, 78-79

Breast pump, 30

Breasts, leaking, 28

Bright, Susie, 238–40

Bureau of Maternal and Child
  Health, 78

Caldicott, Helen, 150

Car payments, 199

Car seat, 31

Career
  having a baby and, 40
  see also Work

Certified Labor Assistant, 47

Cervix, dialated, 51, 52, 53

Certified Nurse-Midwife, 47

Cesarean section, 58, 59, 60, 65, 66
  cost of, 46

Changing tables, 31

Channing, Carol, 122

Checks, fictional, 194, 195, 198

Child abuse, 82

Child care, 162, 165, 167
  work site, 159
  see also Day Care

Child care provider(s)
  checking out, 168–69

Child custody
  see Custody

Child Protective Services, 4–5, 23

Child support, 201–2, 203, 211,
  220
  claim to, 37, 38
  welfare subsidizing, 147, 148

Child Support Enforcement
  Investigation Package, 202

Child support issues, 35

Child support orders, 202

Childbirth, 17, 41–67
  basic rules of, 43
  costs of, 46

Childbirth denial, 44–47

Childbirth preparedness classes,
  45–46

Children
  in divorce/family breakup,
    209, 212–17, 221–23, 226
  teaching about sex, 238–39

Children's rights, 101

Cigarettes, 22

Circumcision, 61–62

Civil Rights Congress, 124

Classism, 115

Clothing
    baby, 29–30
    maternity, 25, 31

Coffee, tea, soda, 22

Cohousing, 131

Collection agents, 195–96, 198

Colleges/universities
    choosing, 164–65

Comfort kit, 31–33

Commission on the Status of
    Women, 36

Communal property, 210–11

Community(ies), 123–24
    building, 203–4
    intentional, 130

Community property laws, 211

Community services, 200

Condoms, 32, 81–82

Conservatives, 149, 152

Constipation, 28

"Contract with America," 146

Contractions, 50, 51–52, 54

Co-op parenting, 129–31

Coparenting, 36
    lesbian and gay, 37

Coparents
    lesbian and gay, 35

Counselors, 34, 218

Court orders, 35
    emergency, 207, 208

Court system, 232, 234

Creativity, 183

Credit, bad, 195, 200

Creditors, 193, 194

Crises
    buying time in, 192–95

Crying jags, 24

Cultural influences
    in gender differences, 119–20,
    121

Culture, 232

Culture shock, 70–71

Custody, 153, 209, 212–17
    given to batterers, 37

Custody agreement(s), 216

Custody case(s), 33, 207–8

Custody issues, 35, 226–27

Custody mediation, 212

Custody orders
    emergency, 208

Darden, Christopher, 219

Day care, 139, 159, 161, 170–71
    see also Child care

Debt, 200

Decompensation, 176

DeJong, Wendy, 169–71

Democratic Party, 154

Denial, 179, 197–98

Depression, 176, 178–80, 183,
    188–91

Diapers, 30, 80

Diet, 21, 29, 186, 208

DiFranco, Ani, 160, 236

Discipline, 104

Discrimination, 159–60

Divorce, 35, 36, 155, 156, 192,
    206, 207, 208, 209

and family ties, 153–54
graceful, 225–28
hostility in, 216
money in, 210–12
positive side to, 224–25, 227–28
retaining sanity in, 217–18
supporting children during,
    221–23, 226
Divorce papers, 207–8
Divorced from Justice (Winner),
    209
Doctor, 28, 29, 47, 52
and donor insemination, 36
and labor, 56
see also Obstetrician
Documents
in emergency, 207
in family court, 220
Dolto, Françoise, 98
Domestic violence, 37–38,
    152–53, 207, 217
and child custody, 215
in divorce, 223
Donor arrangements, 36–37
Doulas, 44, 45, 54, 76, 78
cost of, 46
Drugs
legal, 23
recreational, 23
Dunn, Sarah, 194

Eating
during pregnancy, 19
see also Diet
Economic hardship
and family structure, 154–55
Edema, 25

Elías, Anilú, 98–99, 247
Embryo, 21, 22, 24
Emergency action, 207–8
Emergency shelter/food, 199
Emotions, 191
after childbirth, 68–69,
    70–74, 84
children's, 114
in tantrums, 89–92
Enemas, 56, 59
Environmentalism, 151, 152
Epidural pain relief, 42, 48, 54,
    56, 59
Episiotomy, 57, 59
Equal distribution of assets, 210,
    211
Estés, Clarissa Pinkola, 180, 228
Eviction, 193, 194
Exercise, 29, 186
in third trimester, 28

"Familia Nervosa," 140–42
Family(ies), 2, 3, 5, 83
chosen, 126, 240
in emergencies, 208
gay and lesbian, 37, 154,
    155–56
getting help from, 200
homeless, 201
single-mother, 138
Family breakup, 206–28
Family Channel, 1–2
Family court, 33, 36, 153, 219–21,
    233–34
bias against women in, 209
Family law, 33–38, 156

Family law attorney, 36, 207, 216–17

Family law emergencies, 207–8

Family relations
divorce and, 153–54

Family structure, 154–55, 156
alternative, 33
after divorce, 224

"Family values," 6, 135–156

"Family Values" IQ, 135–39

Famous Writers School, 133

Farm, The, 46, 49

Fathers, 83–84
rights of, 36

Feelings of children
affirming, in family breakup, 222–23
see also Emotions

Feminism, 39, 109, 110, 118, 119, 121, 138
maternal, 122

Feminist mothers, 236

Fetal alcohol syndrome, 22

Fetal development, 28

Fetal monitoring, 54, 56, 59, 60

Fetus, 21, 22, 23, 24, 27, 28

Financial aid (education), 165

Financial mediator(s), 211–12

Financial planners(s), 211

Flex time, 158, 159

Food(s), 22, 24
that smell moldy or unappealing, 22
see also Diet

Food stamps, 3, 147, 167, 197, 198, 200, 201

Formula feedings, supplementary, 79

Free to Be You and Me, 122

French, Linda, 207

Friends, 32–33, 123, 125–26
and childbirth, 45, 48
in divorce, 218
in emergencies, 208
getting help from, 200

Furniture, baby, 31

Garage sale, 196

Gas, 28

Gaskin, Ina May, 46, 49

Gatto, Ramona, 232

Gay and lesbian families, 37, 154, 155–56

Gays
coparenting, 35, 37

Gender, 106–22

Gender differences
cultural influences in, 119–20, 121

Gingrich, Newt, 144–49

Goldberg, Natalie, 184

Gordon, Holly, 109–10

Government, 149, 152–53

Grier, Rosey, 122

Guilt, 60, 235–36
working mothers, 160

Headaches, 28

Health insurance, 200

Heartburn, 24, 28

Help
  when under stress, 180–82
  see also Support
High blood pressure, 29
Hip Mama (zine), 1, 6
Home and Family Show, 1, 2, 3
Home birth, 45, 46, 47, 48–49,
  83
  cost of, 46
Homeless families, 201
Homelessness, 192
Homophobia, 115
Homicide-suicide, 179, 181
Hospital births, 48, 65, 66
  cost of, 46
Hospitals, 44, 45, 54
Hot lines, 69, 179, 182, 207, 218
  suicide, 179
Housewife, 158
Husband
  and childbirth, 48
  rights under law, 34–35
Husband-coached childbirth,
  46

Ibuprofen, 23
Immunization, 81
Immunization Decision, The
  (Neustaedter), 81
Indigestion, 24, 28
Institutions
  as enemies, 232
Insurance, 44–45, 200
Ireland, Jennifer, 139
"Isms," 116

Isolation, 75, 125, 202–3, 240
IV, 57, 59

Jambalaya (Teish), 183
Job sharing, 158
Johnson, Lee, 107–8
Joint custody, 212, 213–15
Judges, 209, 216, 219

Kabat-Zinn, Jon, 184
Katz-Sperich, Betty, 61
Kidnapping, 208
Kitzinger, Sheila, 44
Klein, Melanie, 100
Kujichagulia, Phavia, 235

Labor, 28, 41, 50–54, 66
  complications in, 43
  disappointments in, 60–61
  early, 50–52
  end of, 53–54
  medical interventions, 42–43,
    54–58, 60, 65, 66
  pain of, 45
  premature, 25
  transition, 52–53, 55
Labor force
  mothers in, 158–63
Lakoff, George, 149
La Leche League, 78, 94, 123, 124
Lamaze method (Lamaze-Pavlov),
  45
Lamaze training, 41
Lamott, Anne, 70, 245
Landlord, 193–94, 198

Lavender Families Resource
Network, 37
Law (the)
husband's rights under,
34–35
Lawyer, 34, 35, 37
family law, 36
see also Attorney(s)
Layette, 29–31, 32
LeBoyer method, 45–46
Legal advice
with domestic volence, 37, 38
Legal agreements, 35, 36
marriage as, 40
Legal Aid, 36
Legal custody, 213, 214–15
Legal representation
cost of, 208
Legal services, free or low-cost,
207, 208
Lesbians
coparenting, 35, 37
Life
redesigning, 186–87
Lim, Robin, 75
Long-distance companies, 199
Lorde, Audre, 114–15
Low-birthweight babies, 22, 29

McCoy, Cherie, 102–4
Male privilege, 113, 115
Maleness, 113–14, 120–21
Mamatoto, 54
Mania, 176
Manic episode(s), 176, 177–78, 185

Marriage, 156
and pregnancy, 40
Maternal feminism, 122
Maternal rights, 35
Maternity clothes, 25, 31
Maternity leave, 158, 159
Maternity wards, 52
Mayor's office, 200, 201
Mediation, 212, 217, 220
mandatory, 219
things to remember in, 217
voluntary/involuntary, 216
Mediators, 216–17, 220
Medical attention
high-risk pregnancy, 29
Medical coverage, 200–1
Medical establishment, 44, 232
Medical interventions
in labor, 42–43, 48, 54–58, 60,
65, 66
Medication
for depression, 179–80
Meditation, 183–85, 186
Midwife, 28, 29, 44, 45, 52, 54, 56,
60, 78
costs, 46
direct-entry, 47
Midwifery, 46
Millenial generation, 2–3
Miscarriage, 28, 29
Misogyny, 54, 113, 115, 135
Mitford, Jessica, 53, 132–34
Money
in divorce, 209, 210–12
getting, 196–97, 199–200

Mood swings, 24
Moral Politics (Lakoff), 149
Morning sickness, 12, 24
Mother guilt, 60
Motherhood, 74
    oppression through, 236
    as radicalizing experience,
        84, 232–33
    readiness for, 12–17
    reinventing, 2, 7
    resistance in, 232
    work/school and, 157–71
Motheright, Shamama
    (Siobhan Lowe-Matuk),
        202–5
Motheright (party), 204
Mothering
    guerrilla, 231–41
    imperfectly, 242–47
Mothering instinct, 232
Mothering magazine, 81
Mothers
    categories of, 142–43
    in labor force, 158–63
"Mother's Day Maxim" (Adisa),
    237
MTV, 144, 146

Names, 62–64
National Center for Education
    in Child and Maternal Health,
    62
National Mental Health
    Association, 181
National Organization for
    Women, 30

National Organization of
    Circumcision Information
    Resource Centers, 62
Natural childbirth, 41–43
Natural childbirth movement,
    42, 45, 54
Nervous breakdowns, 175–91
    excuses to cover, 185
Nesler, Ellie, 234
Nesting urge, 27
Networking, 128, 159
Neustaedter, Randall, 81
New Age books on tape, 74
Nin, Anaïs, 245
Norwood, Ken, 130
NOW Legal Defense and
    Education Fund, 202
Nurses of St. Vincent, The:
    Saying "No" to Circumcision
    (documentary), 61–62
Nursing
    see Breast-feeding
Nursing pads, 32
Nurturance, 149

Obstetrician, 29, 45, 47–48, 60
O'Donnell, Rosie, 42
Older Mom, 143
Orgasms, 25
Our Bodies, Ourselves, 51
Out-of-court settlement
    child custody, 213–14
    divorce, 209
Overprotection, 234–35

Panic attacks, 176–77

Parentage, claim to, 36, 37

Parental rights
 in kidnapping, 208
 signing away, 36, 38
 terminating, 37

Parenting, 4, 7
 apocalypse, 149–52
 chaos theory of, 171
 co-op, 129–31
 letting go in, 235
 and politics, 149
 single, 36–37

Parenting guides, 3

Parenting mags, 5–6, 141

Parents
 lack of support for, 88
 noncustodial, 35, 213
 not married, 35
 as role models, 118–19
 same-sex, 155

Parents' rights, 101

Part-time schooling, 165

Part-time work, 158, 169

Paternal rights, 36

Paternity, 35, 38

Paternity rights, 201

Patriarchy, 119, 135, 153, 187

Pediatrician, 81

*Penguin Encyclopedia
 of Modern Warfare*,
 232, 235

Perineal massage, 59

Personal resources, 199–200

Philips, Utah, 82, 105, 219–20

Physical changes during
 pregnancy, 24, 25–26

Physical custody, 213, 214–25

Physical health, 217

Physical punishment, 98

Piercings, 27

Pipher, Mary, 110–11

Pitocin, 57, 59

Placenta, 54, 59

Political activism, 132–34

Politicization, 149–51

Postpartum care, 47, 74–76

Postpartum depression, 69, 189

Potty training, 87, 94–97, 102

Poverty, 192–205
 as challenge, 204–5
 quick fixes, 196–97

Poverty consultant, 202

Power struggles, 102, 103

Prayer, 186

Pregnancy, 11–12, 17–19, 39,
 40
 basic rules of, 21
 batterers and, 34
 care for body during, 19–23
 first trimester, 18, 21, 23–24
 high-risk, 28–29
 nursing and, 81
 others' reactions to, 26
 second trimester, 18, 25–27
 third trimester, 19, 27–28
 weight gain, 24, 25

Pregnancy manuals, 15

Premature babies, 22, 29

Prenatal care, 29

Pre/post nuptial agreements, 35
Profet, Margie, 22
Property division, 35
Protecting Your Baby-to-Be
 (Profet), 22
Protection
 court orders for, 207
Protection/overprotection, 232,
 234–35
Prozac, 179, 190, 191
Psychotic episodes, 69
Pubic hair, shaving, 56, 69

Racism, 115, 116
Radner, Gilda, 246
Rage, 97–100, 103, 104
 in divorce, 225–26
Read (Dick-Read) method, 45
Reagan, Ronald, 142
"Reasonable visitation," 213,
 214, 215
*Rebuilding Community in
 America* (Norwood), 130
*Recognizing and Resolving
 Racism* (Kujichagulia), 235
Referrals
 counseling, 180
 doulas, 47, 76
 family law attorneys, 207
 home birth, 49
 lawyers, 36
 therapists, 218
Religious organizations,
 200, 201
Religious prohibitions about
 sexuality, 239

Religious traditions, 82
Remarriage, 154, 155, 156
Resistance, 232
 guidelines for, 241
Resources
 in family breakup, 218
 outside, 199–201
Responsibilities, delegating, 186
Reviving Ophelia (Pipher),
 110–11
Rights
 in childbirth, 65
 of husbands, 34–35
 of mothers, 159–60
 of parents/of children, 34–35,
 101
Robertson, Pat, 2, 5, 156
Romantic life, 237

St. James, Elaine, 186
Sanitary napkins, 32
Sanity
 in family breakup, 209, 217–18
Savings, 199, 200
School
 and motherhood, 163–67
 part-time, 165
School system, 232, 233
Security, 161
Separation anxiety, 87
Sex
 in pregnancy, 25
 teaching children about,
 238–39
Sex stereotyping, 110–11
Sexism, 107

Sexual life, 237

Shambala Warrior Training, 185

Shared Living Resource Center, 130

Shortness of breath, 28

Simplify Your Life (St. James), 186

Single moms, 136–37, 139, 154, 228
  and child support, 201–2

Single-mother families, 138

Single parenting, 36–37

Slacker Handbook, The (Dunn), 194

Sleep, 186–87, 208

Sleep deprivation, 69, 70

Smoking, 22

Soccer Mom, 142, 157

Social science
  family structure in, 153–55

Social Services, 200, 232

Social workers, 4–5, 219

Socialism, 134

Society of Professionals in Dispute Resolution, 211–12

Sons, 112–15, 120–21

Soren, Tabitha, 144, 145, 146

Sounds True Audio, 74

Spanking, 97–100, 104

Spiegelman-Kern, Tamar, 188–91

Spiritual Midwifery (Gaskin), 46

Stacey, Judith, 153–56

Standard of living
  divorce and, 211

Stanford University, 48

Stepfamilies, 155

Stepparents, 215

Stereotypes, 107–8, 116

Stress
  getting help, 180–82
  response to, 176

Stretch marks, 26

Student loans, 195

Sudafed, 23

Suicide prevention hot line, 179

Support
  village of, 123–34

Support groups, 124, 126–28, 129, 218

Support person(s), 59
  see also Friends

Support system
  in divorce, 218

Supreme Court, 219

Taking care of your soul, 12

Taking leave, 235–38

Teen Mom, 143
  see also Unwed teenage mothers

Teen pregnancy, 137–38, 147–48

Teish, Luisah, 183

Temper tantrums, 87, 88–92

Tenacity, 232–34

Tenants' rights, 198

Tenants' rights association(s), 194

Therapy/therapists, 180, 181, 184
  in divorce, 218
  in family breakup, 226
Thomas, Marlo, 122
Toddlers, 87–105
Toxemia, 29
Toxins, 21, 22
Toys, 109–10
Tylenol, 23, 32

Unwed teenage mothers, 136,
  138, 139
U.S. Sprint, 158
Uterus, 28
Utility company(ies), 193, 194,
  198

Vacuum extraction and forceps,
  58
Vaginal discharge, 28
Varicose veins, 25
Village, finding, 123–31
Village Cluster, 130
Violent thoughts, 69, 99, 179, 181
Visitation, 35, 213, 215, 222
  claim to, 37
  court order for, 207
Vitamins, 21, 22
Viveros, Joy, 115

Walker, Alice, 18, 232
Weaning, 87, 92–94
Weaver, Dennis, 203
Weight gain
  in pregnancy, 24, 25

Welfare, 3, 137, 139, 145, 147,
  165, 197, 200–1, 203
  and child support, 202
Welfare mothers, 149, 157
Welfare Queen (Welfare Mom),
  142–43
Welfare system, reform of,
  135–36, 154
Wherever You Go, There You Are
  (Kabat-Zinn), 184
Winner, Karen, 209
Women in labor force, 155,
  158–63
Women's services, 200
Women's shelters, 36–37, 38, 207
Work
  cutting down on, 187
  and motherhood, 157–71
  part-time, 158, 169
  quitting, 160–63
Work-study, 167
Working at home, 161, 162, 163
  cons in, 166–67
Working Mom, 142
Working Mother magazine, 159
Workplace, mother-friendly, 159
*Wouldn't Take Nothing for My
  Journey Now* (Angelou), 236

Your Baby, Your Way (Kitzinger),
  44

About the Author

Ariel Gore is Maia's mom, a writer, an activist, and the editor-publisher of *Hip Mama*, the parenting zine. Raised in northern California by a small guerrilla army of hippies, artists, and rebel Catholics, she spent the years she was supposed to be in high school as an international bag lady traveling through Asia and Europe. She returned to California at the age of nineteen—baby in tow. Following her misspent youth, she earned a bachelor's degree from Mills College and a master's from the University of California at Berkeley's Graduate School of Journalism. Her articles on motherhood and young feminist issues have appeared in *Parenting, Ms.,* and many other magazines and on-line publications. As a welfare advocate she has debated Newt Gingrich on MTV and made countless other right-wing enemies. She is currently fighting the good fight, praying for revolution, pondering the spirituality of caffeine, and working on her next book.